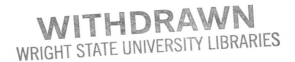
Music and Meaning

Opening minds in the caring and healing professions

Mary Butterton PhD

Musician
and
Senior Registered Practitioner
with the
British Association for Counselling and Psychotherapy

Mary Butterton

Radcliffe Medical Press
Oxford • San Francisco

Radcliffe Medical Press Ltd
18 Marcham Road
Abingdon
Oxon OX14 1AA
United Kingdom

www.radcliffe-oxford.com
The Radcliffe Medical Press electronic catalogue and online ordering facility.
Direct sales to anywhere in the world.

British Library Cataloguing in Publication Data

A catalogue record for this book is available from the British Library.

ISBN 1 85775 817 X

Typeset by Aarontype Limited, Easton, Bristol
Printed and bound by TJ International Ltd, Padstow, Cornwall

Contents

Foreword

What a fantastic subject for a book! We have had so many books on the meaning of life and the meaning of love, but few have attempted to unravel the meaning of music.

Music, of course, like life and love, means many different things to many different people. Just as a particular personality might be abhorrent to some but a potential life partner to others, so it is with a piece of music. A recent study showed vandals 'running scared' when Delius was played over a neighbourhood shopping precinct's music system. They couldn't bear the sweet modulations of that composer's *Walk to the Paradise Garden*. Yet to others, myself included, it is a beautiful piece of music. Likewise, I might easily not appreciate some of the music at the top of those vandal's hit lists. And that opens up a whole other area – the behavioural effect of music. In the late 1950s several American States banned rock and roll for 'inciting riots'. On that basis, they should have banned Stravinsky's *The Rite of Spring*, which provoked a huge disturbance at its Paris premiere.

Although the elusiveness of music's meaning is part of its wonder, the publication of *Music and Meaning* is especially timely. Despite overwhelming evidence that learning a musical instrument develops areas of the brain that help school children with other subjects, music education has suffered severe cut backs throughout the West. As a result, a whole generation has grown up knowing little or nothing about some of mankind's greatest achievements.

Along with countless millions, my life has been immeasurably enriched by music and I can't imagine existing without it. By drawing attention to the immense power of music to literally transform people's lives, *Music and Meaning* could not have arrived with better timing.

Julian Lloyd-Webber
January 2004

Preface

This book has been written from my own experience and life-long curiosity about what music has meant for me and for other people. Music certainly had meaning for other people, as I observed from my home life where my brother sang, and I was aware of its meaning for other people by closely observing my fellow students and tutors at the Royal Scottish Academy of Music in Glasgow. But, talking about what music meant in those days was felt to be unnecessary – one just experienced it. The world of psychotherapy opened up this territory for me.

When I finished at the Royal Scottish Academy of Music I taught in schools and lectured on the appreciation of music for over 20 years. During this time I became further fascinated at how the form or structure of a piece of music could be built up by the class members by asking them to write down what they felt about a particular passage of music. We would find agreement on the broad categories of feeling, such as rising tension or energetic bursts of strong sound. However, beyond these broad categories of agreement on loud and soft, or tension and release, the consensus broke down. The particular fine-grained feelings, such as moments of happiness or sadness, were found to be very different for each class member. In other words, what the fine feelings meant for each person in the class was a very individual experience. People experienced music differently. It was then that I realised that the meaning of music had everything to do with an individual person's life experience – who they were as relating persons in the world.

In later years, when I became involved in the world of counselling and therapy, much of the work done and the thinking around it was about meaning for the client and also for myself. In psychodynamic therapy there seemed to be a link between the psychodynamic processes which are to do with the relationship between client and therapist and the musical process of listening to a piece of music and responding to the ebb and flow of sound. There is a dynamic relationship between client and therapist, as between the listener and his or her music. They seem to occupy the same dynamic field of flowing motion. I next became particularly interested in the fine timing of flowing motion in both disciplines and I also observed layers of process in both fields.

In my own personal psychotherapy some years ago, words eventually became unavailable to me. I was in a wordless dynamic flowing interchange with my therapist. This was to be in a non-verbal or pre-verbal inner place in my mind. One of the only ways I could begin to articulate the quality of feeling was through a description of a piece of music which I then shared with my therapist. In this process I had discovered music as a rich medium of non-verbal and perhaps pre-verbal communication.

I had always been aware of music as a non-verbal communication with many layers to it but the content was veiled and mysterious. I had not thought of asking what a particular passage of music really meant for me. I had not articulated what was special for me in the music. This book is an attempt to draw back the veil a little on this area of meaning for the listener to music. The understandings of what might be going on are assisted by current enquiries, findings and linkages between the disciplines of philosophy of music, neuroscience, developmental psychology and writings in psychoanalysis. Any such understanding of what music means for the listener must, in this present day, be informed by such new and exciting interdisciplinary enquiry. This book is only a beginning.

Acknowledgements

Because the core of this book is interviews with 15 individual persons, I am deeply indepted to all of them for agreeing to take part and allowing us a glimpse into their inner worlds.

I would next like to thank Professor Stephen Pattison for his unfailing support from the very beginning. I am also very grateful to Antonia Murphy, Sue Philips and Penny Hayman, three friends from the world of psychotherapy, who encouraged me from the beginning of the project. I would like to thank Margaret Wilkinson in particular who has been there for me throughout the writing with her strong support.

I would like to remember my brother Hugh Anglim who used to claim that he taught me all I knew about music!

Grateful thanks are due to CS Nair and Annapurna Gautam for welcoming me into the Hindu Community in Derby and helping me to understand something of their culture and music. Wajiha Mohammad is due a special thank-you because she started out as a facilitator of the interview with Safiya and ended up contributing most interestingly to the conversation! Throughout all the writing, Maggie Pettifer of Radcliffe Medical Press has been there for me with her kind help and support and I would like to thank her for this. Finally, I would not have written this book in the first place without the unfailing support of my husband, Harold.

To my husband, Harold, for his love and care

To Music

Thou holy art, how oft in hours of darkness
When life's encircling storms about me whirled
Hast thou renewed warm love in me and gladness
Hast thou conveyed me to a better world
Unto a happier better world

Oft hath a sigh that from thy harp strings sounded
About me breathing sacred harmony
Revealed a joy, a heav'nly bliss unbounded
Thou holy art, for this my thanks to thee
Thou holy art, my thanks to thee.

Introduction

This book is an invitation to the reader from 15 individual music lovers to share in their journey of understanding something of what music means for them. They each took part in a project which asked the question 'What does music mean for you?'. Their insights and discovery of meaning for each of them has involved bringing to words or making verbal what until now has been private, non-verbal and held in their unique experience of performing or listening to music.

Although music is universal what it means for the individual person is a largely unexplored field. The main difficulty seems to be in the area of language. What words can be used to answer the question 'What does music mean for you?'. The person is being asked to describe in words the non-verbal experience of music. Listening to the people interviewed in this book, it is clear that this question opens up the part of the brain to do with feeling and sensation. The conversations begin to come alive, as it were, when the subject of the interview gets in touch with these deep areas of the brain which are then processed in words.

The meaning of music becomes more clear for each person interviewed as each tries to articulate aspects of their felt emotional journey through life. Musical associations with memories of significant relationships and the unique qualities and intensities of these relationships are some of the experiences described. Other experiences, such as music being a direct emotional holding for the listener or practitioner, are also talked about. Music begins here to open up the door to an encounter with inner experience not usually brought to conscious articulation.

In general, to have the experience of music is enough for many people. It is like an internal mirror secretly reflecting back to ourselves who we are and how we relate to others in the world. However, if we begin to wonder about our particular choices of music and want to know something more of what might be behind these choices, we are near to asking 'What does music mean for us?'. But how do we set about this task of finding out what music means for us? And what might we gain from this exploration?

Approaching the meaning of music in the way set out in this book opens up for each of us different and richer ways of understanding who we are, were, or might be in the future. Insights from philosophical writings on the meaning of music and modern psychological theories on the origins of interpersonal engagement provide a backdrop to the thinking. The new findings in neuroscience which link with these modern psychological findings of what goes on in the brain are also felt to be important and useful. All these aspects shade into aspects of spiritual reflection for some of the interviewees, and are both exciting and relevant to what music might be about for us.

Taking the risk of speculating on what one day might be hard science, it is suggested here that the shapings of the dynamic patterning in music are an important doorway to what music might mean for us. The patternings which we individually respond to most in music may turn out to be those which we are already orientated to finding in these flowing tones. This might be so not only because of our genetic predisposition but because these sounding shapes and patterns resonate with what we need to experience and re-experience from early intimate attachments. It would seem that in our search for resonant aural shapings in music we reach out to be further nurtured as developing persons in relationship.

Music looked at in this way could be considered as a reference map which orientates us to what is and was deep and true for us in intimate relationships. Further to this we also get in touch with and experience something of the deep truth of who we are as persons in relationship through this aural mirroring which is music. But how can we begin to know this inner dynamic terrain? Where are the signposts to get us started? For example, we need to know more clearly what we are talking about when we use the word music, and we need to begin to understand something of the linkages we make between the aural shapings of music, the psychological shapings of our inner world of feeling and findings in neuroscience.

This seems a large field of enquiry but we know that persons and music are inextricably linked. Music itself is about pattern and flow in tones. For it to be called music, it should make sense in that it should have a beginning, a middle and an ending, a narrative shaping. When we engage with it and are caught up and feel met in some powerful way in these flowing patterns we are refreshed and exhilarated. This special kind of meeting with the flowing tones which is music is explored here and understanding something of this encounter is attempted. Because we are all unique this understanding will be a different experience for each of us, even as we hear the same shapes and sounding textures.

When we say that listening to music is a different experience for each of us we are suggesting specifically that we bring something individual to this meeting with music. This inner personal aspect also has flow and texture and we feel it in our bodies; we experience it physically as well as mentally.

As has already been said, there is a problem with language in all of this as to how to begin to think about it and then to verbalise these thoughts. Of the writers on the philosophy of music who come close to addressing the questions asked in this book, Victor Zuckerkandl[1] and Susanne Langer[2] are particularly important. Zuckerkandl explores music as a flowing phenomenon which exists in the world. He refers to music as motion in the dynamic field of tones. Langer, on the other hand opens up the thinking on the inner personal terrain of our engagement with music by claiming that we bring to music the dynamic structures of our emotional lives. She holds the view that these dense structures of our emotional lives are met with similar dense structures in music. In these dense structures of music we hear particular musical shapes and textures and we are said to resonate with these particular shapes and textures in their varying intensities in a musical passage. According to Langer these flowing shapes symbolise particularly the flowing shapes and textures of the core dynamics of who we are as persons in relationship, the structure of our emotional life. This thinking and that of other relevant musical philosophical positions will be considered further in Chapter 1.

Often, however, we resonate with these flowing tones from a place of such intensity within us that there seem to be no words to describe this experience. This place of intensity or dynamic inner space, according to modern psychodynamic thinking and developmental psychology, is said to have its roots in an awareness of a flowing frame of interpersonal encounter, or attachment, that is, before words were available to us. Listening to a favourite passage of music therefore could be thought of as having an inner experience of a very early developmental phase where feelings and sensations were very intense but we did not have the maturity of language to use words. This aural experiencing of the shapings and patterning of a given passage of music could be described as a matching or overlap of the shapes and textures in music with the felt memory of the shapes and textures of intimacy in interpersonal encounter. The thinking of the psychoanalyst DW Winnicott on 'transitional phenomena',[3] the developmental psychologist Daniel Stern's writing on 'attunement'[4] and Christopher Bollas' writing on the aesthetic experience[5] are relevant here.

However, these experiences may not be immediately accessible to language. They are known and accessible, however, by another route, that is, through sensations in the body. Getting in touch with the context and dynamic shapes of such feelings and sensations in conversation with another can bring back some of the later associated memories which may then be articulated in words.

When we reach words to describe our experience of music either through self-reflection or through conversation with another to assist this self-reflection, we engage with the musical/emotional experience from a different place, that is, from a place of more conscious thought. There is therefore a change or shift in how we see and experience ourselves. We own the experience of our encounter with music more fully, it has more definition when we are able to bring it to words.

However, as has been said above, this memory may or may not be available to words. If there are no words to describe the intensity of musical experience, it could be that the memory of it is held in the part of the brain which communicates more directly with the body and may bypass words. It does seem as if the felt experience of these memories is held in a place in the mind which can be reawakened through musical patterning. The memory is not in words to begin with but in the body itself and felt as sensation. Neuroscience is most active in exploring this field at present, notably in the work of Damasio.[6] Another neuroscientist working in this field is Trevarthen and he is also making important linkages between the disciplines of neuroscience and music.[7]

This book begins to open up these ways of knowing more about our choices in music and knowing more about who we are and how we have developed as relating persons in the world. As a result of such an exploration, we may discover in our particular musical preferences a too narrow taste in music which we may have needed to stay with because we needed to reaffirm safety and security. The reflective process described in the book may encourage the reader not only to be more daring in her musical choice but also more daring in the ways we approach emotional intimacy with others.

The interviewees in this book are all persons for whom music is important and who have been prepared to write about the meanings of their experiences of music. I am deeply grateful to all of them for taking part in this project and allowing us a glimpse into their very personal inner worlds. They show us how very deep meanings in music can be accessed, thought about and in some way put into words.

The book is in three parts. In Part 1, Chapter 1, the word music is defined and clarified and some different approaches to musical meaning are considered. Chapter 2 introduces some modern psychodynamic thinking on the roots of how we engage with others and the world. It explores some of the many layers of human experience with reference to the findings of neuroscience, developmental psychology and writings in psychoanalysis. A developmental outline of who we are as selves-in-relationship from babyhood to old age will be described alongside our development as musical listeners. Our place as persons in a fast-moving modern society will be briefly addressed.

Possible symbolic links between the dynamic patterning or framing of music and the patterning or framing of our emotional lives is introduced. Psychoanalytic linkages with the findings of neuroscience are also touched on.

In Part 2, each of the 15 people interviewed describes what music means for him or her. At the end of each description the thoughts and feelings of each participant are further explored in conversation with the author. A piece of music chosen by the interviewee is then discussed in some depth.

The author's thinking underpinning these conversations is based on modern psychodynamic understandings of early infant/mother and father relationships and the developing patterns throughout life, as well as new thinking on neural pathways in the brain. From this perspective each individual in the project is understood to bring to the telling of his or her experience the mental traces of early infantile attachments. Not only is something of these early feelings and sensations brought into words, but also, the later more developed experiences of growing up are linked to these early experiences of infancy and childhood and patterns of living in intimate relationships are recognised.

As already described above these patterns are most clearly identifiable at transitional phases of life, for example infancy, adolescence, mid-life, etc. These phases reveal issues of anxiety and loss, but may also have been engaged with positively. Music may be seen as an important transitional medium for the interviewee which held her through difficult psychological transitions in her life.

Asking the question 'What does music mean for you?' of people in adulthood, mid-life and older mid-life is also a question about 'What has life and personal relationships meant for you in the past?' and 'What does life and interpersonal relationships mean for you now?'.

The unique stories which unfold for each person in the project have a different quality about them than that of usual conversation and they may also have a spiritual dimension. They reveal a richness of insight and perception which is also new and fresh to them. They begin to see themselves from a different, richer perspective.

Part 3 draws together common aspects of the participants' stories and also notes the differences. There is reflection on how the participants in the project have used their experiences of music to shape their lives. They have allowed us to share in their understandings, in hindsight as it were. How they now use their increased insight and awareness is for each of them to live out.

As we develop through childhood to adolescence, the questions of meaning in life in a self-reflective way arise. 'Why am I here?' 'What is this life of mine all about?' These questions could be said to have a different quality and urgency during the later phases of life than when they first appeared in adolescence. This might be so because each person has more years to reflect upon than a younger person and also they know that there is now less time ahead to live and enjoy this life fruitfully.

In general, the differences in their stories can be understood to be how each has begun to integrate meaning for themselves-in-relationship with others through reflecting on their experience of music.

The last chapter looks at 'Where we have been', 'Where we are now', and 'Where we are going'. An aesthetic transformational moment in the musical experience of the author is explored and some ways forward in research are suggested.

When we listen to music it has the capacity to hold together the complex mixture of who we are as persons in relationship. What this might be about for each of us is each person's story and journey. When we begin to think and put into words insights which previously were unavailable to us, we begin to reach towards new personal horizons and new neural pathways may be opening up for us. From what we learn about ourselves we may begin to live our lives differently in some ways. This book can open doors to this kind of thinking for you.

References

1   Zuckerkandl V (1956) *Sound and Symbol*. Bollingen Series XLIV. Princeton University Press, Princeton, p. 95.
2   Langer S (1953) *Feeling and Form*. Routledge and Kegan Paul, London.
3   Winnicott DW (1993) The location of cultural experience. In: PL Rudnytsky (ed.) *Transitional Objects and Potential Spaces*. Columbia University Press, New York, p. 3.
4   Stern D (1995) *The Interpersonal World of the Infant*. Basic Books, New York, pp. 157–61.
5   Bollas C (1993) The aesthetic moment and the search for transformation. In: PL Rudnytsky (ed.) *Transitional Objects and Potential Spaces*. Columbia University Press, New York, p. 40.
6   Damasio A (2003) *Looking for Spinoza: joy, sorrow and the feeling brain*. Heinemann, London.
7   Trevarthen C (2002) *Musical Identities*. RAR MacDonald, DJ Hargreaves and D Miell (eds) Oxford University Press, Oxford, pp. 21–38.

PART I

Music and meaning

CHAPTER I

What is music?

'A rose is a rose is a rose' or as might be said here, music is music is music.

In Gertrude Stein's famous poetic phrase, the word music could be substituted for rose. This suggests that if you have to ask the question 'What is a rose?', there is a simple answer – the repetition of the word rose – and so it is with music. But there may also be a more complex answer.

EM Foster approaches this complexity in his book *Howards End*. He writes here of Helen's thoughts on leaving a concert she has attended with a group of friends and relations:

> Helen pushed her way out during the applause, she desired to be alone. The music had summed up to her all that had happened or could happen in her career. She read it as a tangible statement, which could never be superseded. The notes meant this and that to her, and they could have no other meaning. She pushed right out of the building, and walked slowly down the outside staircase, breathing the autumnal air, and then she strolled home.[1]

In this passage, Helen is portrayed as attributing meaning to music. For her it is more than a pleasurable experience of sounding patterns of tones and rhythms, it has powerful meanings for her about her very existence. Here we meet an awareness of the complexity of music. We can begin to look at this complexity further by considering some relevant writings on the philosophy of music, from two distinct groups, the realists and the personalists.

The realists

The realist group of thinkers consider that the relationships between the tones which make up the melodies in music already exist in the world, as does the ebb and flow of rhythm. These thinkers maintain that there is 'to and fro' motion in the universe present in different phenomena, for example the sea, or the planets. The collective term for these phenomena is fields. These phenomena are called fields of motion, and the motion of and within the phenomena can be felt, heard and/or seen. For example, the lapping of the waves on the seashore describes the motion in the dynamic field of gravity; this motion may be felt, seen and heard. The sound of wind in the trees describes dynamic motion in the air around us. In Purcell's *Ode on St Cecilias' Day 1692*, the poet Nicholas Brady writes:

'Hark, Hark each tree its silence breaks
The Box and Fir to talk begin.'

However, this is a *poetic* idea of conversation between trees through the sounding tones made by the wind in the branches. In other words Nicholas Brady is describing dynamic motion in the 'to and fro' movement of the sounds heard in the wind. Important also in this passage is that these sounds are said to relate to each other here; there is, as it were a conversation.

A more modern philosophical view from a realist perspective is that of Victor Zuckerkandl. Writing in 1956, he describes music as 'motion in the dynamic field of tones'.[2] Here we are introduced to another dynamic field, that of the sounding tones themselves.

To put this more simply he holds the view that there is 'to and fro' dynamic motion in the sonic field of tones, that is, there is motion between the tones themselves. However, Zuckerkandl in another book, *Man the Musician*, writes that these musical tones are made by humankind; they do not exist of themselves.[3] How these tones relate dynamically to each other will be considered later in this chapter.

Another group of thinkers, the personalists, hold the view that not only are human beings essential to the making of music, as we generally understand it, but also that the shaping of our emotional lives can be heard in the patterns of flowing tonal relationships. Their thinking will now be briefly considered.

The personalists

These thinkers take the view that for music to be music, human beings must shape the sounding tones to make music. This much Zuckerkandl agrees with. Susanne Langer belongs to this group of personalists and she writes in *Feeling and Form*[4] that in this process of experiencing music we hear sounding symbols of the structures of our emotional lives. Put more simply, her notion of structures in music incorporates shapes and textures of sound which resonate with the structures, the shapes and textures, of our emotional lives. These are heard by us in passages of music through a length of time.

For example a passage of music, such as the opening of Brahms' *First Symphony*, could be thought of as ascending shapings in sound which form a presenting structure. There is increased tension in the texture of this strong sinewy, striving shape. It reaches towards a powerful climax before fragmenting into hesitant, plaintive conversational woodwind writing. According to Langer, such a shaping in music, the rising muscular tension of the texture, could be said to be symbolic of the shapes of rising tension within our inner world of thoughts, feeling and sensations – our inner experiences, from the past and in the present.

To explain more clearly, the shapings and textures in the *field* of our inner world of feelings, thoughts and sensations are said to be reflected in the shapings and textures in the *field* of music. This will be explored later in more detail. However, having introduced humankind into this discussion brings us nearer to the experience of music and what this might mean. To open up this topic we will look briefly at how we as human beings might perceive music.

What of meaning in music?

When we play or listen to music we experience a very rich personal sensory, emotional and intellectual phenomenon, each in our unique way. We experience music, as it were, through layers of perception within ourselves. One layer could be concerned with the shape and felt sensation of the flowing sounds heard. Another layer could describe experiencing the dynamic tensions in the tones and rhythms of music, as well as an appreciation of the flow and dramatic narrative. A further layer, and the one most particular to this book, is what music *means* for any individual.

In *Howards End*, EM Foster understood these levels of human perception. He writes of the members of the party attending the concert referred to above as follows:

> It will generally be admitted that Beethoven's *Fifth Symphony* is the most sublime noise that has ever penetrated into the ear of man. All sorts and conditions are satisfied by it. Whether you are like Mrs Munt, and tap surreptitiously when the tunes come − of course, not so as to disturb the others; or like Helen, who can see heroes and shipwrecks in the music's flood; or like Margaret, who can only see the music; or like Tibby, who is profoundly versed in counterpoint, and holds the full score open on his knee.[5]

Each layer of perception described here is to do with the listener's experience of dynamic shapings in tone and rhythm, which reach her from outside her body. In receiving these dynamic shapings, she resonates with them. This would be like Mrs Munt tapping in response to Beethoven's rhythms; or Helen, who projects imaginatively into the presenting shapes and textures. We already know, however, that Helen goes further than these projections to reach the layer of meaning in her life. From the passage quoted earlier, she is said to have these deeper thoughts as she leaves the concert hall by herself. Tibby is intrigued intellectually by the music and studies objectively the shapings and textures in the counterpoint. Margaret is said to 'see only the music'. This is an enigmatic statement. One wonders if Margaret, through this musical experience, is in touch with depths of her inner world which reach beyond words, beyond projective images.

These perceptions can be about everyday life experiences, or they can engage with memories, that is, contexts and structures of past experiences, or all of these phenomena together. In hearing and receiving these dynamic shapings the listener experiences music.

It must be added that not only might these complex layers of music be experienced in any combination or singly, they may also be encountered all together in a rich interwoven aural experience.

Having suggested that there may be more to the experience of music than initially meets the ear, other aspects of how music is experienced will now be looked at.

Music to my ears!

What sounds as music to one person is experienced as noise by another. Personal preference could be put forward as the reason for this state of affairs, but this side-steps the problem rather than engaging with it.

Personal preferences in music rest on how we experience it. From simple observation, the rock concert listener is obviously caught up in the excitement of sound. He or she is responding to a particular sounding phenomenon, the dynamic shapings of sound which is rock music. Likewise the chamber music listener or the audience member at the 'proms' is personally engaged in different dynamic shapings of sound. These shapings, however, are said to ebb and flow in this dynamic field of tones, and more needs to be said about this field and what it is.

The dynamic field of tones

Zuckerkandl has described music as 'motion in the dynamic field of tones'. This field of motion he names as the 'Third Stage',[6] an area not identical with the human psyche nor identical with the physical world. This 'Third Stage' is said to stand in the relationship of the primary to the derivative like a central flowing core encountered through the physical world and the world of persons.

But we as persons encounter this field of tones through listening to music and the tones come to us from without. These tones are shaped into what we know as music by persons. The music is of these persons, composers. This 'Third Stage' then is the domain of tones and is also the personal. Music therefore has that about it of human interpersonal motion and communion.

According to Langer, this musical communication or dynamic motion in and through music between persons describes intensities, shapes, textures and patterns in the tones and rhythms in music, which have been arranged in a relational context. When we listen to a passage of music we are said to experience a relational context.

To explain these terms further, intensities refers to degrees of striving from one tone to another. In the fourth movement of Sibelius' *Second Symphony*, there is a slow build up of great intensity before the statement of the broad, majestic first subject or theme. It is suggested here that the magnificence of this theme is in part due to the deliberate build up in degrees of intensity of the climbing phrases immediately before. The shaping of the repetitive rising scale-like writing, and the increasing thickening of the instrumental texture along with the unsettling punctuated rhythms, form a powerful intense shaping. This powerful architectural build up reaches its climax in a freely flowing powerful melody. There has been a sense of striving and completion or resolution which makes emotional sense. Langer writes that, 'The symbolic power of music lies in the fact that it creates a pattern of tensions and resolutions'.[7]

It may be noted here that there is no description of what the composer himself might feel. It is a view held by the author that such a description of Sibelius' own particular feelings would be mere speculation; unless, of course, he had let these feelings be known verbally. What we do know and hear are the shapings of feeling of Sibelius which he has framed through tonal relations and communicated to us.

Returning to the reader's understanding of the relational context which frames the tensions and resolutions in music, this phrase, the relational context, needs more explanation. However, without going further at this point into the technical musical detail of this important phrase, a brief explanation may bring some clarity as to its particular meaning.

A relational context here means that the tones and rhythmic pulses are drawn towards each other in a musical framing which, through its rhythmic and tonal tensions, seeks a resolution, a sense of completion. One overarching way of describing it, is to say that the relational context has a beginning, a middle and an end. In the Sibelius example above, the beginning of this particular relational context is quiet. This is followed by a tremulous, slowly building tension through the middle section reaching towards an ending or resolution in the broad majestic theme.

However, not only do different types of music, such as rock music or chamber music, occupy similar but different shapings in this dynamic field of music but the listener or performer of rock music or chamber music each occupies an inner world of similar but different shapes of mental personal dynamics. We will now consider further this inner world of persons-in-relationship.

The dyamic field of persons

We have discussed shape and texture in the opening of Brahms' *First Symphony*. According to Langer's thinking each listener might agree on the striving shape and sinewy texture of this passage of music, but what these shapes and textures mean in the world of inner feelings will be different and particular to each listener. Further to this, a musical passage or temporal sounding of tones may be thought of as a condensed symbol of many experiences for the one listener.[8] This means that more than one feeling or sensation may be heard simultaneously. The music may be heard as sweet, beautiful and also deeply tragic and painful at the same time.

These individual experiences or personal dynamic feelings or sensations within each of us are different in nature and unique to each person. Each one of us may project her unique feelings, thoughts and sensations into the same piece of music and have quite different internal mental experiences even though we do have the same *basic* brain structure. What is different in the brain structure for each person is the wiring of the neural pathways.[9] When we encounter music these different inner mental pathways and connections are to do with who we are as persons, as experiencing listeners or performers, at the time of listening to or performing the music.

We are now moving towards talking about two larger categories, the dynamic *fields* in which these shapings of intensities, textures and patterns occur. There is the dynamic field of music which reaches us from outside our bodies and the dynamic field of persons, with their inner mental shapings, their internal worlds. These two dynamic fields overlap in the experience of listening to or performing music.

The overlap of dynamic fields

As an experiencing person we each mentally occupy constellations, or gatherings, of dynamic shapings in our internal mental world; the world of thoughts, sensations and feelings. When we engage with others verbally and non-verbally, we enter other people's internal worlds or dynamic constellations. These inner worlds or constellations and our engagement with other peoples internal worlds will be discussed further in Chapter 2. For the moment it is enough to state that these interpersonal encounters with other people are in constant dynamic flux between us and them.

For example, I may feel irritated with a colleague, but over a period of time, I do not remain irritated to exactly the same degree. I either feel more angry and irritated or I feel less so. This dynamic flux between me and her is another way of saying that we are in interpersonal dynamic relationship. Our relating is a living changing state, and this living changing state is experienced within the dynamic field of persons. Feelings and sensations are recognised as important within this dynamic field of persons.

Dynamic motion in music

With regard to music, Zuckerkandl[2] has defined this same kind of flowing movement or flux within music itself as motion in the dynamic field of tones. When one tone meets another in a melody it is governed by the position of the most important note in its constellation or pattern of tones. Other tones are said to relate to this important note. This anchor note is known as the key note or tonic in whichever tonal pattern or key is established. Even if the music is said to be atonal, that is, not having a recognised key, Zuckerkandl believes that a tonal pattern will be established whatever. This might be, for example, through the rhythmic repetition of one particular note which becomes heard as the most important anchor note and a constellation of tonal relationships is aurally experienced around it. However, what must not be lost sight of is that Zuckerkandl also holds firmly to the fact that persons create the tones of music. Tones do not exist as music independently in the universe.

When we experience music therefore, we are in the overlap or meeting place of these two dynamic fields, the personal field and the musical field. However, just to say that we experience music is in itself too broad a statement. How we experience music needs further clarification.

Two ways of addressing this issue are to think about music objectively and subjectively. To consider music objectively would be to study its form and structure out there, as it were, as Tibby studies counterpoint in *Howards End*. Or, music could be approached subjectively, that is, to encounter it in our inner world of thought, sensation and emotion. Helen and perhaps Margaret in *Howards End* would be said to encounter music subjectively. We will now look further at the experience of music from an objective view and then from a subjective perspective.

The experience of music looked at objectively

Music can be considered objectively in order to distinguish it from noise. John Sloboda defines music as 'the creation and resolution of motivated tension'.[10] This suggests that, to be called music, this sounding phenomenon should have a beginning, a middle and an ending, a narrative shape. Other prolonged sounds such as the ticking of a clock or a prolonged monotone would not therefore be considered as music according to this definition. However, the lapping of the waves on the seashore, which in its 'to and fro' motion is very listenable to, might be considered as music here. One can hear the tension in the rise of the wave and the resolution when it falls; but if music is to be the creation and resolution of motivated tension, the question arises as to whether the rise of the wave can be described as truly motivated. If so, who is doing the motivating?

This is a difficult area. We do not create the dynamic of the lapping of the waves. This is of a different kind of order but it exists in the world not outside it. This dynamic ebb and flow of the waves is considered by Zuckerkandl to be derivative of the motion in the core of life itself.

He writes:

> There must be a layer in which all things have their roots; the tones, so to speak, activate this layer and thereby bring us closer to the roots of things ... Mystics speak of a place where 'all things are together' ... This source is also the domain of tones.[11]

We will consider this thinking more fully in a later chapter. For the moment, musical ordering will be thought of as specific to human action and be framed within a humanly intended dynamic plot. That is, music will be considered from the point of view of having a beginning, a middle and an end.

This comes near to the notion that for music to be called music it needs to have a dynamic narrative in sounding motion in which humankind is involved. It may be, also, that it is this human dynamic shaping in sound which we respond to most immediately in music. This leads on to what this dynamic story, which is music, might mean for you or me, the listener.

At this point it should be made clear that the use of the term dynamic story or narrative does not mean that any external programme is necessary for music to be music. The dynamic story referred to here describes the tonal and dramatic tensions in the ebb and flow of the sounding tones and rhythms which frame a beginning, middle and ending. There may also be an external story, as in opera, but the dynamic story or narrative referred to here is found in the ebb and flow of the tonal relationships.

However, this dynamic story shaped by the composer in the tones, rhythms of music and patterns of sound in music meets another dynamic field, that is, the inner world of the experiencing listener or performer. This meeting can be described as experiencing music subjectively.

The experience of music looked at subjectively

Modern psychodynamic thought takes the view that the aspects of an individual human being, her brain, her intelligence, feelings and bodily sensations, these aspects of each of us, which are the building materials of our human story, are in internal dynamic encounter with each other. Not only are these aspects in dynamic encounter with each other internally, they are also in dynamic encounter with the world around us and the persons with whom we engage. In our living we respond through our minds and bodies to the outside world. Music is a flowing sounding dynamic phenomenon in the world and we respond to it through the meeting of these two dynamic fields, that of the field of being a relating person and the field of relationships within music.

When we begin to take the view that our minds and bodies are in dynamic relationship with music, Susanne Langer's thinking on the meaning of music becomes important. In *Music and the Emotions*, Malcolm Budd considers fully Langer's idea that music is a symbol of the structure of our emotional lives. He also explores further her idea of music as an 'unconsummated symbol' of the structure of our emotional lives.[8] By naming it as an 'unconsummated symbol' Langer tries to make it clear that music does not symbolise the *nature* of any particular feeling an individual might experience, that is sadness or joy, etc., but she claims that music symbolises the *structure* of any feeling. The structure is its shape and texture, the *ways* in which feelings are expressed, for example in a kind of surging way, or a rushing way, or in a halting way, or in an explosive way. Different feelings can be expressed under the one structural heading; anger for instance can be described in a surging way; joy can be expressed in a surging way

This truth can be observed in that people respond differently to the same passage of music. For example, the main energetic theme, which is a strong dramatic musical statement, heard at the beginning of Beethoven's *Fourth Symphony* can be experienced with feelings of joy, or triumph, or with angry rage. This is also an example of one dynamic musical pattern or shape carrying more than one projected feeling simultaneously. Put simply, it is the structure or dynamic shapes within music itself which we meet in the musical encounter and then we as individuals supply the particular sensations or feelings.

We may be guided of course in some music by comments made by the composer, for example the *Eroica Symphony* of Beethoven. There are many verbal clues given by the composer about the nature of this music, but we still put our own complex feelings and sensations into the dynamic shapes and textures which Beethoven presents us with.

Langer writes that the shapes and intensities in music are symbols of the shapes and intensities of the dynamic life of our feelings and that when we listen to music we resonate with these shapes, these dynamic journeys within music.

In this book these theories are important as applied to the personal stories told by the members of the project. They provide us with insights into how each engages in particular interpersonal relationships at a deep level and how music frames the shapes and contours of their individual thoughts, feelings and sensations for them. In Chapters 3 to 12 each member of the project describes in turn what music means for each of them and these thoughts and feelings are then briefly reflected upon. Individual stories begin to unfold of how these particular musical shapings have become deeply important for each interviewee. The possible meanings of the shapes and contours each person hears in music will begin to be heard.

References

1   Foster EM (2000) *Howards End*. Penguin Books, p. 47. (First published in England in 1910 by Edward Artnold.)
2   Zuckerkandl V (1956) *Sound and Symbol*. Bollingen Series XLIV. Princeton University Press, Princeton, p. 95.
3   Zuckerkandl V (1973) *Man the Musician*. Bollingen Series XLIV 2. Princeton University Press, Princeton, pp. 14–15.
4   Langer S (1953) *Feeling and Form*. Routledge and Kegan Paul, London.
5   Foster EM (2000) *Howards End*. Penguin Books, p. 64. (First published in England in 1910 by Edward Arnold.)
6   Zuckerkandl V (1956) *Sound and Symbol*. Bollingen Series XLIV. Princeton University Press, Princeton, p. 142.
7   Langer S (1953) *Feeling and Form*. London, Routledge and Kegan Paul, p. 371.
8   Budd M (1985) *Music and the Emotions*. Routledge and Kegan Paul, London, pp. 104–20. (For a full account of Langer's theory of music as a condensed symbol.)
9   Damasio A (2003) *Looking for Spinoza: joy, sorrow and the feeling brain*. Heinemann, London, p. 32.
10 Sloboda J (1985) *The Musical Mind*. Oxford University Press, Oxford, p. 22.
11 Zuckerkandl V (1973) *Man the Musician*. Bollingen Series XLIV 2. Princeton University Press, Princeton, pp. 41–42.

CHAPTER 2

Who do I think I'm listening to?

In the last chapter we briefly considered music and its meaning within the tones themselves, and how music could be said to have a deep dynamic structure which we may experience within many layers of our listening to music. For example, Mrs Munt's tapping of the fingers while listening to Beethoven's *Fifth Symphony* at a concert would be experiencing music at a level which engages the physical body in movement. Another layer would be the imaginative layer, like Helen who sees pictures in the music, or there is a layer which associates music with particular people and places. However, there is yet another layer which can be described as the seemingly unfathomable place of flowing sensation of the 'away from' and 'towards' dynamic motion that Margaret in *Howards End* is described as experiencing when she is said to 'see only the music'.

This chapter will explore some of these layers of human experience further by referring to modern research done in neuroscience, developmental psychology and writings in psychoanalysis. There will then be an outline of a developing sense of self and music and the chapter will finish with a brief consideration of the swift-changing violent world for the person under 40, as today's global society is a powerful backcloth against which any experience of a modern sense of self and self-in-relationship must be lived.

Layers of human experience informed by neuroscience, developmental psychology and psychoanalysis

Mrs Munt's physical response to the rhythmic motion in the music can be thought of as the person experiencing bodily feeling and sensation. Looked at from the perspective of the neuroscience of human persons, Colwyn Trevarthen describes three systems in the brain which evolve in dependence of each other.[1] They are particularly concerned with music here. The first one is the Intrinsic Motive Formation system the IMF, and he has identified it in the brain's reticular and limbic core. He writes that it is a coordinator and regulator of movements and their prospective and sensory control. One could perhaps hold the view that this basic human movement system is a link with Zuckerkandl's idea of motion at the core of life itself.[2] It is what human beings do with the 'away from' and 'towards' motion in the world.

Trevarthen's findings are to do with the brain and body of the human person especially the newborn infant. In the brain of the newborn baby he finds as fundamental this 'Intrinsic Motive Formation' system, the IMF. It is a dynamic motion system, a flowing frame we seem to be born with. It determines both expressive and receptive states and it contains generators of dynamic tension. He then identifies a second system as the Intrinsic Motive Pulse system, the IMP. This is a body-moving, rhythmic and emotionally modulated system, and is seen as the 'agent' of the IMF system, the first system. We now have identified for us, systems, which measure the motion of our human lives from the earliest stage.

One important aspect particularly relevant to this book is that Trevarthen believes that the contemplative listening aspect of music gains its primary values from standards of emotive power and harmony and beauty that are set within the receptive architecture of the basic IMF system, the first system. This means that we are born with the potential to hear and appreciate beauty and harmony, but whether we develop this capacity of appreciation must depend on later nurturing factors. Trevarthen is especially interested in the *active* dynamic musical interchange but he has outlined the *contemplative* listening aspect of his work. This implies that much more detailed research on the receptive side needs to be undertaken.

Returning to Trevarthen's thinking on the origins of musical interchanges he holds the view that many of the structures in the human brain are present in the embryo. They are important in early infant communi-cation and are formed in the brain long before the cerebral cortex begins to be formed. The IMF system and the IMP system are two of these structures. We now know something of the origin of Mrs Munt's tapping fingers, but there may also be much more meaning here for Mrs Munt which has not been explored.

Trevarthen goes on to write that the IMF system is the first one established and its neural anatomy persists throughout life in the brain stem, basal ganglia and limbic structures as a third system, the Emotional Motor system, but the *listener's* music owes its origin to the IMF system, the first one. It will be clear that the systems identified are each dependent on the one before and the whole structure of the brain is built on such complexity.

As human beings in the womb we first experience bodily sensation and feeling, and these are our first experiences of dynamic motion. The experience of rhythmical music engages us from our first beginnings from this dynamic place within us, a non-verbal place. Every infant therefore has these 'musical' roots in his or her physical human nature and structure. From a wider adult experience, Damasio[3] identifies how the brain is engaged in listening to music. Along with Trevarthen he also identifies a layer of 'away from' and 'towards', a dynamic pulse in the biological beginnings of all living organisms. I will consider further his writing on the adult experience of listening to music in a later chapter but, for now, we will explore further this non-verbal place within us.

The non-verbal experience

In the reflections and memories of the interviewees on music in this book, the most difficult experience to articulate in words belongs to the sensation of flowing shadowy layers of 'away from' and 'towards' in the brain and body when listening to music which is important for them.

This is an experience in listening to music which seems to be beyond clarity of description in words. The listener who experiences this deeply satisfying flowing layer from time to time may struggle with meaning here. The content material seems to be beyond words and is sometimes called a spiritual experience. This could be connected with a memory of a recent religious experience but it is suggested here that he may also be reaching into a pre-verbal trace of such an experience in the psyche, that is, before words were available to him as an infant.

This listener may be encountering in his or her non-verbal or pre-verbal experience something of early encounters with beauty and aspects of containment and reverie with mother or carer from a time of infancy in his or her life. From a spiritual perspective the flowing experience may also be understood as a glimpse of something of God eternally present and holding all things together. The religious person might also consider that this glimpse of God may be a sign of the existence of the eternal God who he or she will encounter when this temporal life is over. Generally, all that the listener can manage to articulate is that he or she is enthralled and held by a flowing sensation of great beauty.

From another perspective Michael Tippet, the composer, would seem to be recognising the experience of a deep flowing backcloth to music when he writes of it as feelings perceived as the sensation of flow.[4] In *The Musical Envelope*,[5] Le Court goes further and makes a link with this sense of non-verbal flow with the psychoanalyst DW Winnicott's thinking on mother and child when he describes this flowing experience as if caught up in a lulling sensation of weightlessness while being carried by mother. This linking of the inner flowing mental state of how one feels held by music to Winnicott's ideas of being held in a loving holding reverie by mother firmly connects the experience of music to the experience of the young baby in the infant/mother relationship.

From his experience as an analyst in the consulting room, Christopher Bollas has written of the traces in the adult patient of very early infant dynamic flowing experiences of reverie with his or her first carers. He also writes that when any of us as adults meet such experiences in art or music we may feel a sense of transformation just as we did as infants with our first carer.[6]

Further recent refined studies of this developmental stage in infant relating with mother tell us still more about the content of this early experience of flow, but in terms of active dynamic interchange rather than a state of stillness between mother and baby. In this active dynamic interchange Trevarthen has observed and measured 'proto conversations' as if these exchanges were verbal conversations, but through such non-verbal sounds as squeals and gurgles, and bodily movements between infant and mother.[7] Also Stern, the developmental psychologist, describes these dynamic and relational shapings, the squeals and gurgles of the infant through a passage of time, as having the properties of musical terms such as crescendo, decrescendo, sudden stopping, surging, etc. He names these shapings of feeling as 'vitality affects'.[8]

Having looked very briefly at very early states of infancy and music we will now consider how we develop as selves and selves-in-relationship with music.

Developing senses of self and music

The sense of self in the infant

We start life as baby musical listeners and active participants in the forms of feeling and sensation in the womb, and from these first experiences, if all goes well, we are born into a place of further containment and developing trust with mother, our first carer. We have already 'taken in' while in the womb the modes or ways of being with her, the 'vitality affects', of surging, rushing, crescendo, decrescendo, fading, etc. which we hear and experience in our developing bodies and brains. We hear and experience her heartbeat and the flow of blood around us, and her moments of stillness through the quieting of her heartbeat and maybe a flowing sensation of just being held. We hear outside sounds too, her voice, her singing and music, along with other noises.

Trevarthen writes that the newborn absorbs this mood or atmosphere of a mother's gentle sounds as he or she listens to a peaceful musical recording, perhaps, or the hum and rhythm of convivial conversation.[9] When we are born into this musical to and fro with mother we seek sympathetic engagement with her, partly because she can *transform* our lives in that she makes us more comfortable and removes anything which causes pain and irritation.

Mother sings and communicates with us. This is done through soft cooing and lalling sounds, a reflexive enjoyable musical melody. There are also moments of quiet reverie with her as we are held gently in the arms of our mother or our first carer. All this takes place along with the tactile experience of her in the first weeks and months of life.

Musically, this is the time of the lullaby. This soothing experience is recognised by us as babies and we are temporarily calmed. Shortly afterwards, this musical engagement develops even further into a more developed two-way vocal exchange with our mother and other carers.

Psychologically, we, in this place as infants relating to mother and father or their substitutes, establish a blueprint, as it were, for all other kinds of intimate relationships throughout our lives. However, from a psychoanalytic perspective Bollas writes that we also begin to experience mother as an object who can transform us, that is, our physical and felt world, as we first grow in loving attention with her. He holds the view that when we hear great music which carries the maternal properties of holding and containment we reach back, as it were, to the hope of such wonder and transformation.[10]

The first two years of human development is the frame for all further growth in our sense of self-in-relationship . It is also our musical and artistic babyhood and is the cradle of sensitivity to touch, sound and colour. We first experience these artistic forms in this place of early infancy. But we do grow and move on.

This growth even from infancy involves a period of transition which returns throughout life as we grow up and grow older. These periods of transition are the times of managing loss as well as gain. For example in babyhood we must give up being physically carried by mother like a little king or queen in order to find out more about the interesting world around us, especially when it is through the back door and into the muddy garden.

We also begin to re-experience periods of transition at times of personal crisis and we may be reluctant to move forward with our lives because change involves some kind of loss as well as gain. However, we really do need to risk the challenge both physically and in terms of personal relationships in order to grow and develop. We will now consider briefly these later signposts of growth.

Our sense of self-in-relationship as a toddler onwards

As we become more mobile through crawling and toddling we grow in the direction of becoming more autonomous little people while still in relationship. We are then immediately confronted with the dilemma of holding on to mother or letting go of her for short periods. If all has gone well enough in the early meeting with our carer (mother or mother substitute), in that we trust her more than we mistrust her, we are better placed to dare to let go sometimes and explore the world. Musically, we might dare to make loud banging sounds on a drum or bang saucepan lids together, which might startle us but nothing much else happens, the world does not collapse. Mother of course might divert this exploratory banging as it might be doing her head in!

From a therapeutic perspective, this early experience of choosing loud exciting noises, managing to tolerate them and perhaps enjoying them might encourage a sense of achievement, a sense of 'I can do this'. This early rewarding experience might be valuable in later life when, for example, we choose to listen to exciting music after a diet of holding containing music especially after a time of severe loss. Our choice of louder more exciting sounds might describe our capacity to move on with our lives when we begin tentatively to explore again new sounds and experiences.

Child's play in peer groups describes the information on the next signpost. In this play age of four to seven, there is identification with parents in fantasy and the child explores who she is in terms of sexual identity. Conscience makes an appearance. Outgoing initiative is balanced against feelings of guilt. Musically, this is the time of confidently joining in the class percussion group and enjoyment in turn-taking (which we have learned much earlier in games with mother) and making group music. Also there is great delight in making noises of all descriptions.

At the school age of about 5 to 11 there are no major physical changes to contend with and school work, interest in the external world and social relationships are important in the child's neighbourhood. This is a time of school achievement and competence and at the same time feelings of inferiority. In terms of music, at this stage children often learn to play a musical instrument and gain pride in their achievement and appropriate mastery. Musical games in the classroom are also enjoyed.

At adolescence and young adulthood at roughly 12 to 17 or 18 years, or even until 20 or 30 in this changing world, interest in sexuality is given highest importance. There is a drive to establish more fully a sense of I and I-in-relationship and this is a powerful struggle. There is a recapitulation of the early ways of being in infancy and early childhood, a reworking of issues at those times which were not and could not be resolved because of physical and emotional immaturity, for example intense loving feelings with a sexual aspect around the age of four or five when the young child is 'in love' with the parent of the opposite sex. The reworking of these feelings as teenagers and in our early 20s with peer partners uncovers once again issues of trust and mistrust in interpersonal relationships. Further to this there are issues of control and a sense of self-worth with regard to sexual and social roles to be worked through. All of these issues, along with emancipation from parents, make this a difficult time for the young people and their parents.

Music is very important at this stage and in the Western world the wild dance and pop music engaged in may be linked to the two-year-old's banging of the drum and the message to the parents 'How much can you take?'.

As we grow through the personal and interpersonal confusion of this period and apart from the need for self-assertion and rebelliousness in wild kinds of music, sensitivity to beauty of sound and tonal colour are quickly being further developed, and often go hand in hand with the rebellious sounds. How this stage and its struggles are managed paves the way for later more mature adulthood.

There are no major physical changes to contend with at this stage of adulthood, but issues of intimacy versus isolation figure large during this period, as has been said above. Personal involvement and competition and cooperation come to the fore, and supportive partnership is still considered as valuable.

We test ourselves by the effective contributions we make to others. We do this through friendships, love, sport, hobbies and the capacity to earn money. Partnership, marriage, parenthood or being alone are all states that exist in adulthood and have to be negotiated. This negotiation depends on how we have managed the transitions from the earlier states of being in relationship. When problems arise in personal relationships or we meet serious loss through divorce or the death of someone close, we may have enough resources to grieve for a time and then slowly move on in our lives. If the loss is too traumatic we may need some therapeutic help. Listening to or playing music, however, may be a solace at these times of loss, allowing us to be held and nurtured while we slowly come out of the grief of loss. Particular pieces of music may be especially significant for us as individuals and seem to speak directly to us at these times.

Midlife is another time of crisis and transition. Here we slowly become aware of the time left before death and are perhaps spurred to do things we really want to do in the time left. Some people change careers and are given, as it were, a new lease of life. But it is also a time of reflection and self-absorption and some people gradually come to a place of acceptance of who they are and that they are not going to be prime minister (male or female!!!). Grandchildren become important here and caring for others in the family takes up any spare time. Spiritual questions such as 'Who am I?' gain prominence and we may reassess ourselves here also.

Musically, we know what we want to listen to and value it for its aesthetic beauty as well as its capacity to reawaken memories of events and persons important to us. This reminds and consolidates for us who we are and were. We may join in choirs, or play in music groups, or become passionate about particular forms of music like jazz, folk, or classical music and we identify with it as *our* music.

Retirement is often marked by the ending of money-earning work. The crisis of transition here is about 'Who am I as I reach towards the end of my life? Have I done enough with my life for it to have been worthwhile or is there more for me to learn and creatively engage in?, Can I be of help to others now since I missed out on being prime minister all those years ago?'.

We might conclude that it is much more effective to be of help to others locally than to have been the latter. Also 'Can I still grow and learn how to be in relationship?'. There may be grandchildren to enjoy! Many retired people also give their time to local committees, such as being a school governor, or freely give their expertise to a charity or a community project. It can be a very busy and fulfilling time, but it will also have its quieter moments.

Music can be of great importance at this time of life when our free time may be used more reflectively. If we have played an instrument we may join a group of musicians and make fine music together or sing in a choir. We may also listen to music and reflect on our lives and enjoy the beauty of sound that is still there for us. All of these activities can continue into older age as the oldest interviewee, the 100-year-old Reverend Reg Dean, will show us. But what more do we know about the interviewees?

The interviewees

We turn now to the persons who are interviewed in the coming chapters. Each of these persons is unique but they also belong to different groupings in society. In these groupings there are differences in age, culture and nationality. These differences are easily observed from the outside, as it were, but there are other differences too. Each person is unique in his or her inherited characteristics. Each has been born into a different arrangement of family relationships which have influenced who he or she was as an infant and who each has become as a teenager and adult. As a result of heredity we bring into the world a combination of strengths and weaknesses of each of our parents and some inherited traits are more powerful than others in contributing to who we are. This combination of traits is part of our nature. There is, however, another part of who we are. That is, how we have been nurtured. As has been said above, each person is born from a sexual meeting of the mother and father from whom we inherit a set of personal characteristics, but how this mother and father or substitute mother and father engage with the newborn infant will have had a powerful influence on the baby's physical and emotional growth in the early months and years. For example, was mother, in particular, emotionally strong and confident and also gentle and calming? And was father supportive of mother and also protective of her, sharing the stress of a new baby in the household?

If 'yes' is the answer to these questions it sounds an ideal environment for the new baby. But it is just that, an ideal. Most parents engage emotionally and physically with the infant in a 'good enough' way for the infant to grow and thrive so that there is no lasting emotional damage done to the infant's physical or emotional world. However, what an infant hears, sees and processes in these early stages of their existence is beginning to be understood more clearly through the writings of DW Winnicott, Daniel Stern, Colwyn Trevarthen, Antonio Damasio, Christopher Bollas and others writing in this field of early development and experience. These writers attend to the dynamic interactions between mother and infant and mother, father and infant.

The developmental writing of Daniel Stern and Colwyn Trevarthen in particular gives weight and clear measurable evidence to some of these early family dynamics. How the infant negotiates these early family dynamics is being studied. How the baby and carers together create a feeling-and-sensation dynamic blueprint which is hard-wired in the brain, as it were, is being researched now in this exciting field of modern early infant neuroscientific and human development. This blueprint within our minds is unique to each of us but it may still be capable of change.

If we widen the influence on the creation of this dynamic inner blueprint to include not only mother and perhaps father figures as first carers, the inherited traits from both parents and the influence of other family members and the larger community, we can begin to recognise the wonderfully rich dynamic relational influences on the malleable early blueprint within the baby. We are all truly unique and interesting people. Having stated this, we must consider an even wider frame than that of the family. This would be the frame of present day society.

A larger sociological perspective

Even though we start in a small unit of infant/mother relationship, people aged under 40 experience a very different world in terms of society out there than that experienced by the above writers on neuroscience, the philosophy of music, developmental psychology and psychoanalysis, and this author.

Large shifts in the behaviour of society have markedly impinged on the personal individual development of who we are as growing relating persons. Young people and growing adults have much more freedom in the present day but also more anxiety perhaps about who they are, that is, their identity as persons. They also have more difficulty in understanding what relating to others means for them. They are thrown back as never before on themselves for answers to the questions of existence and how to have good enough relational lives both in intimacy with other persons and with the world at large.

There is a big problem here in that the more ordered family life of 50 years ago has given way to many forms of relational living. Among the many variants are traditional marriage with more choice to end it through divorce, and partnerships in the form of monogamous serial relationships, same sex relationships or the life of living alone. These are only some of the possibilities.

One of the most important aspects of living in the twenty-first century is being a member of a world society which is at the moment fragmented and threatened by terrorism. This is a frightening backcloth to any form of living.

Hopefully, younger people under 40 have companions and relatives who from time to time support and help them over this difficult terrain. Music will have been there all the time throughout their lives and their choice of listening may reflect their even more uncertain journey of what it means to be a human being-in-relationship in the twenty-first century. The basic blueprint of relating is still the first two years of life and we hope that there is enough of a sense of trust in their basic sense of self and self-in-relationship to hold and sustain them with music alongside as their non-verbal companion. In the following chapters we will turn to the stories and conversations of our interviewees.

References

1   Trevarthen C (1999) Musicality and the intrinsic motive pulse: evidence from human psychobiology and infant communication. *Musicae Scientiae*. Special Issue 1999–2000. The European Society for Cognitive Sciences, Belgium, pp. 155–211.
2   Zuckerkandl V (1956) *Sound and Symbol*. Bollingen Series XLIV. Princeton University Press, Princeton, p. 95.
3   Damasio A (2003) *Looking for Spinoza: joy, sorrow and the feeling brain*. Heinemann, London, pp. 102–3.
4   Tippett M (1989) Art judgement and belief: towards the condition of music. In: P Abbs (ed.) *The Symbolic Order*. The Falmer Press, East Sussex, p. 41.
5   Le Court E (1990) The musical envelope. In: D Anzio (ed.) *Psychic Envelopes*. Karnac Books, London, p. 213.
6   Bollas C (1987) *The Shadow of the Object*. Columbia University Press, New York, pp. 13–40.
7   Trevarthen C (2001) Intrinsic motives for companionship in understanding: their origin, development, and significance for infant mental health. *Infant Mental Health Journal*. **22**: 95–131.

8 Stern D (1995) *The Interpersonal World of the Infant*. Basic Books, New York, pp. 56–7.

9 Trevarthen C and Malloch S (2002) Musicality and music before three: human vitality and invention shared with pride. *Journal of Zero to Three*. **23**: 10–18.

10 Bollas C (1987) *The Shadow of the Object*. Columbia University Press, New York, p. 17.

PART 2

The project

CHAPTER 3

Interview with Maeve

Maeve is a retired art teacher who paints and writes for *Open House*, a lay Catholic journal. She also acts as a guide to the Burrell Collection in Glasgow and sings in a liturgical choir while (as she says) waiting patiently for one of her family to produce some grandchildren!

Maeve's writing

A few years ago I was taking part in a discussion as a volunteer worker with a group of prisoners' wives. There were a number of set questions, one of which was, 'Did you have any particular role model apart from your parents between the ages of seven and eleven?'.

I was surprised to find that while others happily chatted away about favourite teachers, supportive aunties and even helpful Guide leaders, I couldn't think of one person who was constant and continuous during that period of my life, including my parents. A combination of war, a variety of schools (mostly boarding schools) and a certain amount of ill health made a disaster area of those early years. What I had assumed to be a rather privileged upbringing was really a fragmented and deprived one. Having absorbed that little revelation, it occurred to me that, of course, music had formed a sense of continuity for me.

I came from an extended family where most people played the piano with varying degrees of ability and sang regardless of ability. The first boarding school I attended had lots of would-be pianists and violinists, a school choir and the usual cycle of seasonal hymns including plain chant. Choirs were very important to me at school. Listening to those national anthems at school during the war made a strong impact upon me. The Polish girls were particularly good. They played some Chopin and Paderewski's *Minuet* as a matter of national pride but one girl played a very muscular Brahms' *Rhapsody Number 2* – stirring stuff! For years I thought Brahms was Polish!

I do believe that music at this stage came to represent a great deal more than mere enjoyment. It was the link with that other world I had left behind. It was a comfort. It was a language I understood. I was learning to play the piano and I was seven and a half.

A couple of schools and a year or two of illness later my father died and what was left of the family moved to Glasgow. The plentiful supply of home-produced music dried up. It is difficult to remember how much effort and dedication it took to hear any music in those days. I would scrutinise the *Radio Times* at the beginning of the week for favourite pieces on the Third Programme concerts and catch Jack Jackson on Radio Luxembourg.

I had developed a good ear for picking up themes and background music from films that I might only have seen once. Unfortunately, this prevented me learning how to actually read music and I became adept at 'playing by ear'. I can still see one of my teachers turning the music back a couple of pages and saying 'start from there'. I hadn't a clue. She took it as a personal insult!

My appetite for music was voracious, indiscriminate and largely uncritical. From early exposure to piano music I was acquainted with Beethoven sonatas, lots of Chopin, Mendelssohn, Schubert, Brahms, Mozart and sundry light classics. There was also Gospel singers, jazz, Gershwin, Gilbert and Sullivan, pop music and the Irish melodies of Thomas Moore. Irish emigrant songs lent a good bit of meaningful heartache to the return from holidays with relatives in Ireland.

Teenage years became quite lonely and I began to extrapolate life from music rather than the other way round. I imagined a future fitted to the great romantic themes and soaring orchestral dramas that I was now beginning to know. Real life, when I finally met it, was a bit of a shock, and sex was a definite disappointment. Boyfriends would be infuriated by my total absorption in some favourite piece of music on the Third Programme. My mother advised me to keep men and music well separated.

My mother had a rather odd attitude to strife within the family and would not tolerate fights that are usual in most families. However, we all had our own tastes in music and whatever fighting did occur did so on those grounds. Strangely my mother seemed to find that quite acceptable. The message seemed to be that music was worth fighting over while other things were not.

Later I married a man who had little or no feeling for music, I felt obscurely that our capacity for disagreement would be limited. In fact it merely limited our scope for mutual enjoyment and for many years I heard very little music at all. When I had my own children, I found that I distrusted the part that music had played in my life and didn't want them wallowing in any emotional sublimation quite unfitted to the modern age. I felt that I had been emotionally retarded.

It would be dishonest to say that music did not enrich my life enormously, but I know that my attachment to it was out of all proportion to the rest of my life. And yet it was not an addiction. I could do without it and did for long periods. Life was just very drab without it. I felt that my own children needed a balanced ordinary life – to be the same as everyone else rather than some weirdo with ridiculous tastes.

Conversation with Maeve

MB: It has always struck me Maeve that music has been very important for you.

Maeve: Yes, it still is.

MB: You talk about continuity in music but not in your experience of growing up. This suggests to me that there might be some confusion for you about how others might have related with you or did not relate with you. I wonder if you felt you were not quite sure where you were with people while you were growing up?

Maeve: Well, I went from school to school and during that period there was no continuity. There was no one person I related to (including my parents) . . . a rather deprived childhood in that sense.

MB: And you learn best, don't you, through continuity . . . how things are done, and how people relate . . . this is part of how you learn about relationships.

Maeve: Also you have to learn very quickly when you go into a new situation, how to cope, how to manage the situation.

MB: But often you deal with the situation but do not attend to what is happening inside you.

Maeve: I think that most people would now agree that a child being shunted from one boarding school to another is not advisable. It has a lot of bad emotional effects. You make a set of relationships and then you are rooted up and sent into another set of relationship challenges.

MB: And there is no time to process the grief from the first lot of ended relationships.

Maeve: And there is also the fact that I was off school ill for a year and a half.

MB: That was a long time.

Maeve: And when I went back to school it was a different school.

MB: It was quite chaotic for you in many ways.

Maeve: It was very chaotic, and there was also a war on!

MB: I wonder if you felt that music helped to join up your life in some way . . . was able to hold you in some way?

Maeve: I always loved music . . . music was always there . . . and I had a good memory for music so I could carry a lot of music in my mind.

MB: And you talk about how when you were at boarding school music was a link with what was out there at home . . . the ordinary things out there . . . and it also held for you perhaps that sense of belonging in your family. There is a sense of wistfulness associated with how you talk about music, a kind of lostness somehow?

Maeve: The blitz was going on. You didn't know what was happening. I remember a conversation I overheard outside the dormitory. A woman was talking to the head teacher ... she was giving an account of all the places that had been flattened by the bombing over the previous weekend. Two of the places Gourock and Greenock were where my family were ... she had come back with my mother. I didn't know that until I looked out of the window the next morning and saw my mother walking up the drive ... so she was safe.

MB: That must have been very frightening and upsetting for you. You talk about your illness.

Maeve: I had a peculiar sort of pneumonia, silent pneumonia. I was walking around with this undiagnosed. I went home for Christmas and my mother decided there was something wrong with me and called in a consultant. He diagnosed this and I was then in bed for several months. I had to learn to walk again when I got up. This of course was pre-antibiotics, pre-penicillin ... but I got better!

MB: How old were you then?

Maeve: Nine and a half, I think.

Maeve went on to talk of the years between nine and a half and 13 when her father died. She was two years in another boarding school which was very strict and she was only allowed to talk for three and a half hours a day. All her schools were convent boarding schools where she writes that the Catholic ethos was very much about subduing your own instincts.

Maeve: They didn't even encourage very close friendships. This was about the fear of sexuality as we know now but we were totally unaware of that then. The nuns themselves were not encouraged to have close relationships with anybody ... but maybe they hoped we would all become nuns eventually ... so we were brought up as mini nuns. One school in particular prized silence ... it was the rule. You kept silent from getting up until 8 a.m. breakfast. Then I became ill again first with diphtheria and then chickenpox. So I was taken home and I was off school again, this time for a term.

MB: So your whole schooling was interrupted ... not only your sense of learning and continuity of learning but your relationships with the other girls was very disrupted. But then of course your father died. So what of the family then, your two brothers and a sister?

Maeve: We all had a very disjointed childhood, all of us, because we were away at school.

MB: So when did you see them?

Maeve: We saw each other during the holidays ... we were all at home then.

MB: I wonder how you feel about all of this now. I wonder if there is any anger around about all that happened?

Maeve: Anger was not an option. It would have achieved nothing. I feel I've had too little anger in my life for too long.

MB: It's very understandable isn't it. It seems that anger was not an emotion available to you at that time. You were also in a series of schools where what's inside you, your feelings, are not attended to.

Maeve: There was very little anger ... you accept things as a child. And I've accepted things most of my life ... I couldn't even afford to show anger as a teenager ... I've often thought that there are people who cannot afford an emotional life. Full stop! Anger appeared very much later in my adult life and not particularly related to this period.

MB: That sounds as if you couldn't afford an emotional life?

Maeve: I couldn't afford an emotional life.

MB: That sounds a scary thing for me to ask of you? To think about?

Maeve: I would still say that the whole family is ... semi-detached ... that's just the way things are ... and some are quite happy to be semi-detached.

MB: That's right ... it's how you deal with who you are within a particular family?

Maeve: Yes ... sure.

MB: You say a bit of you refused to take in formal music teaching? I wonder what that was about?

Maeve: It could have been about the upheaval when my father died.

MB: That could have had a powerful impact upon you?

Maeve: Yes, yes ... everything circled around him ... he was the kingpin ... he was a doctor. At that time his calls and business were very central ... certainly if the patients came to the house, which they did.

MB: So that was part of your life too ... there were patients coming in and out ... so you had to be quiet?

Maeve: You had to be quiet and you never had to repeat anything you heard in the house.

MB: So the silence comes in again?

Maeve: Oh yes, totally.

MB: It is interesting this veil of silence that follows you through your life ... at different schools ... at home ... because this is how things are. It seems lonely perhaps?

Maeve: Yes, I would have preferred to have had a more articulate background but there was the Irish element also. When you went to Ireland everybody talked ... all the time. It is said that in Ireland you talk in self-defence ... also there were the songs that they sang there. All the very beautiful Thomas Moore ones . . . but they also sang *Come back Paddy Reilley.*

MB: They sang about close relationships which perhaps you didn't experience personally?

Maeve: Those kind of relationships didn't apply to our part of the family.

MB: But you met it when you went to Ireland. In Ireland you met the opposite of silence, this wonderful bubbling sense of life . . . so Ireland is very important to you?

Maeve: Well . . . I did say when I was 15 or 16 that I was not Irish . . . I was Scottish. So I made this decision . . . but Ireland has a great attraction for me.

MB: I'm sure it does . . . I'm sure its better than silence. You say that you almost constantly lived in music in your teenage years rather than in real life. Can you say something more about this?

Maeve: After the death of my father I was suddenly at a day school which was another new experience. My mother was distracted with other things, the rest of the family. My older sister and one of my brothers were going through a period of upheaval and my mother didn't cope very well and they didn't cope very well and I was pottering along at school. I would be 14.

MB: A very vulnerable age.

Maeve: Very vulnerable in the sense that when I chose my school subjects, I chose art because the school had a nice art room at the top of the building and you could go and hide yourself away there.

MB: So the most important subjects for you were artistic?

Maeve: No . . . because I've never been an artist . . . I liked writing . . . but there was a lot more freedom in the art room. Freedom had now become important to me. My mother didn't know anything about this until my results came out.

MB: You mean that your mother didn't know that you had chosen art?

Maeve: Ah . . . yes! She didn't know.

MB: And what was her response?

Maeve: She was quite horrified. I did go to art school but I wasn't all that enthusiastic about going. I would have preferred to join a newspaper.

MB: Maeve you write that your attachment to music cut you off from aspects of the rest of your life and that you distrust that part in music. Can you say a bit more about this?

Maeve: I think I wasted too much time listening to music and it was important to me out of all proportion to the practical elements of my life. I think I would have been better served if I had spent more time drawing, for example . . . spending more time on things that would have been of use to me to make a living later on.

Listening to music is such a private thing that too much listening can prevent you from engaging with life or people. Music feeds into your imaginative life ... but it's not real life!

MB: It is interesting that the music you have chosen is about other people joining together and making music ... there is a connection between music and people which you have discovered. This is a place where you can meet both.

Maeve: There is also the spiritual aspect here. I associate some choir singing with church ... the spiritual aspect that can't be put into words, like that other art in churches such as stained glass windows and woodcarving. I think artists, wood-carvers, craftsmen and craftswomen convey the essence of spirituality rather than academic theological argument.

MB: I'm wondering if music and a sense of belonging in community are very important for you. Would that be right?

Maeve: Yes I think so ... I think that is spiritual.

MB: Now the music which you have chosen *Nkosi Sikelela* is the South African National Anthem and it is a prayer to the Holy Spirit. What is it that so moves you in this prayer.

Nkosi Sikelela   **Composed by Enoch Sontonga (1897)**

God bless Africa,
Let it's banner be raised;
Hear our prayers and bless us
Descend, O Spirit, descend,
O spirit descend
O Holy Spirit.

Maeve: I didn't know it was about that.

MB: That's very interesting in itself ... It carries something for you that words don't need to explain?

Maeve: Right ... it's the music not the words ... maybe it reaches back to when I was very young and listened to all those different national anthems at school. I was conscious of a deeply emotional reaction from my school friends around me ... the Polish and the French anthems in particular ... I am very susceptible to national music. Freedom has been the leitmotif of the twentieth century from two world wars to sixties individualism and that would have affected me.

MB: Do you know what that susceptibility is about?

Maeve: It's the choir ... it's the nationalism ... the freedom aspect, and there is a rawness and vulnerability in it. I was recently in Poland at an ordination of a

Catholic priest and the national anthem was sung by adults and children together ... and I wish to God I felt about my country something of what they feel about theirs ... there is an intensity and a loyalty that is very appealing.

MB: So in this piece of chosen music Maeve ... what do you resonate with?

Maeve: I think there are several strands which come together for me. First it's the choral singing and next in this piece there is a rawness, a freedom, and it sounds so natural. It also has yearning in it. It is unashamedly emotional. It starts as a call in the early morning, building up to an intensity of group national feeling. For me the feeling defies analysis ... it is carried in the music which has the capacity to reduce me to tears. I access this space inside me through music ... I would take this to my desert island!

MB: Thank you very much Maeve.

CHAPTER 4

Interview with Keith

Keith was born in Cornwall and educated there and in Wales. He taught for 40 years in school, a college of education, a polytechnic and a university. Since retirement he has been heavily involved in the University of the Third Age and is now the Chairman.

Keith's writing

The beginning was the soprano voice. Ours was not a particularly happy home but people usually rallied for Christmas. I recall my mother calling me into a kitchen unusually rich in cooking smells with the words 'Come quick! An angel on the wireless'. It was Isobel Baillie in a pre-Christmas broadcast of the *Messiah*. We possessed an organ and later a piano. My parents came from Cornish Methodist families and there was a great deal of hymn singing, my father later moved on to *O Isis and Osiris* making great play with the last low F. I begged to be allowed to 'learn the piano', finally succeeding only to be moved away to another town after three months. The lessons did not recommence. 'Well, he's learned the notes' they said. Music did not feature in the secondary school curriculum in wartime Cornwall and it was not until university days that I really 'heard' recorded music, went to a live concert (Verdi's *Requiem*) and realised that music was playing a substantial part in my life. National service in Berlin completed this undergraduate 'education'. My first opera was *Tristan und Isolde*, Dietrich Fischer Dieskau was 'in residence' in the city . . . . London for the next 50 years provided the 'postgraduate' courses.

My main interest was in music as the supreme non-referential art, the embodiment of the abstraction which I saw as the main element of modernism. 'All art aspires constantly towards the condition of music.' Pater's[1] insight seemed to lead the way to the great twentieth century explorations and, paradoxically, to my own fascination with the frontier between words and music. While seeking an escape into a region which was pure structure and form with no clogging reference to the 'real' world, I was held back by the 'word' and the infinite possibility of its 'meaning'. I had no interest in 'word music', a little more in writers who described musical works (Foster, Thomas Mann), and was most intrigued by those who adapted musical form to literary artefacts (Eliot) and went furthest into the unknown territory where the word 'became' music. In the Western tradition Joyce is supreme. After early experiments such as the Sirens chapter in *Ulysses* he embarked on the final 'noise and silence' of *Finnegans Wake*. Some literary theorists hail this as the *only* book as all we can do is 'read' it – just as some feel that all we can do is 'listen' to music. I am reminded of a Third Programme series by Hans Keller in which the announced analyses of Beethoven's late quartets were wordless. Fragments were juxtaposed, repeated, transformed and so on.

The literature/music analogy does not, however, quite hold in my case. I am not a writer, and certainly not a composer, but I did continue to play the piano after those first few lessons and, late in life, was lucky to meet an exceptional teacher. She respected my decision not to prepare for examinations and together we have explored a wide range of music ranging from Schöenberg (I studied a piece to play to my literature group who were reading Thomas Mann's *Dr Faustus*) to more familiar fare. After retirement I took up another instrument. The oboe was a false start. I could not get to physical grips with the diminution required and went to the other extreme with the more embraceable 'cello'. Learning not to achieve but just to 'do' was a kind of liberation, and if the experience has sometimes been more notable for its masochistic pleasures, I have learned finally to 'listen'. This can be disconcerting. At first I only heard the lower string lines (wonderful in *Die Walküre*, by the way!) but I find that the ear (even the ageing ear) can be trained. This dimension of my relationship with music is vitally important.

Perhaps in some way I am still in my mother's embrace although I am only conscious of spending most of my life trying to escape it. She did sing. Cornish girls in the early part of the century sang regularly in chapel choirs and I remember her telling me of the agonies of holding on to the seemingly ever rising soprano line in the Hallelujah chorus. I still hear my father's resonant bass, and on a recent visit to Newlyn the air seemed full of those male voice choirs which 'brought the roof off' the grim chapels. I went to a family wedding some years ago and, after a tremendously loud rendering of a tenor solo while the couple were in the vestry, my cousin leaned back from the pew in front and said 'He gave it bell-tink'. I have no idea of the linguistic origin of this. I also remember coming home from that first Verdi's *Requiem* in Liverpool and my friend saying, 'I like the loud bits best'.

In the end, perhaps the 'loud bits' are drowning out the world. Music is an 'escape' but in the end the word may be supreme and:

'. . . tears shall drown the wind'.

Conversation with Keith

MB: Keith, in your writing there seems to be a note of sadness, of disappointment about not having had a more formal musical education?

Keith: That's certainly true . . . I deeply regret this . . . I think I would rather have had a musical career than anything to do with literature.

MB: So music is more than just important for you?

Keith: I would have liked it to have been more important in a real sense, that's why I have striven to make the connection between words and music in my life. My career has been in words and I have always longed for the other and somehow to bring them together . . . the wordlessness really. I didn't write in my piece that I had a very powerful soprano voice as a boy but it was completely untrained and I can remember the neighbours saying to my mother, "O you must get that boy's voice trained". But no one was interested and nobody did it.

MB: That's the sadness that comes through?

Keith: It is a sadness. I've always loved singing and I had a passably light tenor voice. When I started teaching, the school I taught in had a very accomplished choir. They travelled to Germany to broadcast and I sang with them. I sang the tenor line but I had a tonsillectomy in my early 30s, was very ill and I never sang again, until just when I retired I joined a madrigal group. I found them over-accomplished . . . they could all sightread. They kept saying "You'll pick it up Keith" but nobody taught me how to do it . . . so my attempts at singing have been a great sadness.

MB: You go on to tell of a time when Walter Pater's phrase had a very significant meaning for you, 'All art aspires constantly towards the condition of music'.[1] Could you say a bit more about this condition and how it is that this phrase has such importance for you?

Keith: It's because he opened up the way to thinking about non-referential art . . . I've always striven to inhabit a world where works of art are abstract above all else. (I've always loved abstract painting.) . . . and I've always striven for a world which didn't have a referential meaning. That's why I have so embraced some of the structuralist positions as a teacher of literature because quite often their analysis refers only to the relationships between the words within a poem or a play. They don't refer to the outside world at all.

MB: Michael Tippett, like you Keith, also considers this phrase of Pater as non-referential to the outside world . . . but he goes on to claim that a work of art's meaning, especially music, has something to do with the inner world of feeling and emotion.[2]

Keith: Yes . . . I think formalism in the arts allows for a relationship between one's inner world of feeling and emotion with the work of art without reference to the life we're living in the external world and I think that's the attraction of abstraction in painting, sculpture, literature and music. Pater has put this very neatly into words. A lot of modern art, particularly in my field of literature, has striven towards a move away from a situation in which the artist can be asked what the artefact means in terms of the outside world and can only say what it 'means' in terms of the world he or she has created. This seems to be a natural state in the world of abstract music. When a musical composition is described in programme notes, the written word cannot mirror the experience of the creator or listener.

MB: Keith you seem to be fascinated with this frontier between words and music. Can you say a bit more about this?

Keith: Yes, I'm a modernist and I've always been interested in twentieth century writers who explored this relationship between music and language.

I invited Keith to say a bit more about this relationship between music and language. He went on to describe the evolution of words and music to include 'word music' a kind of sound patterning, for example the nonsense rhymes of Edward Lear, 'Twas brillig and the slithy toad', etc., and then on to EM Foster writing in *Howards End* of Helen's description of a shipwreck in Beethoven's *Fifth Symphony*. This he described as an external picturesque approach.

The last stage and the most significant for Keith is the writing of James Joyce and the novel *Finnegans Wake* in particular. The most important aspect of this work for him is that the work has no meaning at all in referential terms and therefore it is the nearest in relationship to music. He says that all you can do is read it and experience it. I asked him if he could say more about this experience of *Finnegans Wake*. He continued . . .

Keith: It is an endless delight. First you have to get rid of all negative expectations of what a novel should be; what it should do; you must just go with it. It is primarily for some people a rhythmic experience . . . it is I suppose literally a breakthrough in that English is not enough. Many other languages are drawn in. The sounds are filled with German, Sanskrit . . . it is a structure which . . .

MB: Which moves?

Keith: Well that is a key word of course because the book begins with the word 'riverrun' . . . it flows . . . and the end of the novel which is not only the death of the character but the death of 'the novel' itself is about the river running into the sea . . . the last word of the book 'the' joins up with the first 'riverrun'. Joyce himself suggested humorously that only an insomniac would read this book. It is a night book . . . a book of the unconscious. It does the impossible if you like. It brings the unconscious into language . . . it is a musical flowing rhythmic experience. And so it seems to me that it is endless delight . . . it constantly denies reference to any meaning and in that it remains supreme.

MB: What about the title *Finnegans Wake*. What is wake here?

Keith: Well, it is a very good example of what I've been talking about because it cannot be pinned down to a specific meaning . . . it could be 'wake' as in Ireland, the celebration after a funeral. It could be an injunction, an imperative asking Finnegans to wake up. The explorations of meaning are many, that's why the absence of the apostrophe is so vital! You can't read it in the sense of reading to establish a settled meaning.

MB: Another possible meaning could be a sea image, the wake, the flowing after.

Keith: Yes, it has all sorts of possibilities. In a way you need a group to read it, the ebb and flow . . . people pouring in their ideas.

MB: Even the language you use is very fluid.

Keith: Yes . . . it's a wonderful novel.

MB: Can we turn to something else you write about with enthusiasm, your taking up a musical instrument later in life? Is there any room for suggesting that, at last, music had become word for you? In other words you began to communicate who you were through music?

Keith: Well, it wasn't quite like that at the beginning. I had always had the piano which didn't quite feel as if I was communicating who I was.

MB: How is it you say that?

Keith: Because with the piano the notes are made for you and you are not creating the whole sound in the same way as, for example, a string instrument . . . I had become very ill and the oboe was suggested but this didn't work for me . . . I felt I wanted to reach out and embrace music through the instrument, and the oboe reed was a diminution, a dilution almost. So the cello seemed to meet this physical need I had in relating to music. It was almost a sexual experience . . . but again it wasn't as successful as I would have wanted, because you can never be really good taking up a stringed instrument so late in life . . . but I very much liked that you made the note yourself . . . there was also an entirely new dimension to listening. I was simultaneously training to be a Samaritan, which is all about listening, but this didn't work out. However, I shall never regret doing the training because it really brought before me, as never before, the art of listening. I felt very guilty about it. I had been teaching for 40 years and I had never listened enough to my students. The combination of the Samaritan training and having to listen to the notes you made on the cello was very exciting and instructive for me.

MB: That would be a really attentive listening?

Keith: Very . . . it was a quite different form of listening . . . you had to listen to the cello with such care to hear if you were playing flat . . . I don't think I ever listened while playing the piano. When I started going afresh to concerts and opera I began to hear stringed instruments very keenly, so since that time, my listening has had an extra dimension. I shall never regret taking up the cello . . . but I wish I had done it when I was seven . . . what a different life I would have had.

MB: Different is the word. There is a kind of listening in depth when you listen to a cello in an orchestral piece . . . you say that your ear has been trained since then. What would you say you hear anew and what might that mean for you?

Keith: I think I hear more accurately and I didn't think that was possible. Now I play in a small group and I am very aware when people are not in tune . . . it's immensely satisfying playing in this group. There are eight of us and we've all had similar experiences, either we have given up playing for years and come back to it or someone has just started the clarinet, for example, and we play together every Monday afternoon.

MB: And are you patient with one another?

Keith: People are extremely patient . . . it is a University of the Third Age class so the whole idea of that is helping each other. Sometimes we break up into smaller groups but mostly we play together . . . so I am extremely grateful for my listening training. Although there are things that defeat me at times and I cannot play them, it is still important that I belong to such a group.

MB: At the end of your piece of writing you describe music as an escape. An escape from where, I wonder?

Keith: I really don't know. Maybe it's life . . . I'm still very uncertain where this quest is leading.

MB: Where might you think it is going for you?

Keith: I think it is a quest for home in some sense . . . we're all seeking a home . . . I haven't found one yet.

MB: Yes . . . can you describe this home?

Keith: It's a return to where one started . . . where one feels physically right . . . physically in place . . . physically less jangled.

MB: Integrated? . . . in tune?

Keith: Yes . . . in tune might be a way of describing it . . . and I think everybody is seeking this.

MB: Yes indeed.

Keith: I have the feeling that musicians, accomplished musicians, have found it . . . they're already there . . . but that might not be right and they may say this is not so. But being in music, like them, seems to me like coming home. Sometimes I feel that I would give up everything if I could just keep playing with that group on a Monday and play for the rest of our lives together. It seems a silly thing to say but for me it's a kind of ultimate. And it's very satisfying.

MB: I wonder if you feel that the experience of playing with this group is almost perhaps pointing to something else?

Keith: Mmn . . . I think it is . . . there is something else . . . when we meet as a group and talk about whether we should have a performance in front of an audience, I don't want to do that . . . that doesn't satisfy me.

MB: That's an 'outside experience' if you like? And what you're talking about is something else? Michael Tippett, writing in *The Symbolic Order*[2] suggests that there is a flow to be found behind music . . . does that have any meaning for you in this context?

Keith: Yes, I think it does . . . perhaps he is saying something about this rhythmic experience . . . which isn't to do with the structure of melody or such which is also satisfying in music. Tippett was a composer and he may have been talking about the creative flow which is the well spring of writing music . . . he may have been talking about his own experience.

MB: Mmn . . . but he does go further to talk about this flow being behind all things.

Keith: Yes . . . I think perhaps he meant this famous term 'the unconscious' . . . and to go back to Pater and Joyce, perhaps if they were to articulate it they would say something like that. A possible aspiration for artists is giving voice to the unconscious to articulate the unconscious which is an impossibility because the unconscious does not have a precise language. Freud commented that the royal road to the unconscious was the dream and to my mind Joyce's *Finnegans Wake* is *the* literary work which comes nearest to expressing this idea. To most people it is joyously meaningless . . . this voice to some people articulates madness . . . but I think that Michael Tippett may have been making the link here to psychoanalysis . . . the talking cure.

MB: I'm interested that you say that . . . because you say above that you are searching for home and home is what we know in some way already from childhood . . . and the 'unconscious' is a very adult concept.

Keith: Yes . . . of course it is.

MB: And to talk of the unconscious presumes the presence of a conscious state . . . but what of the preconscious state of early infancy where as yet there is only a crackling towards consciousness. Given that modern psychoanalytic thought holds the view that we carry traces within us of very early experiences, I'm wondering if there is a link to be made with the TS Eliot phrase 'In my end is my beginning?'. Are we, perhaps, through some kinds of music reaching towards this early state from a more adult place . . . a revisiting?

Keith: 'In my end is my beginning' is of course a quotation from a work with a musical title *The Four Quartets* . . . and perhaps music is a feeding of the unconscious towards this state . . . maybe it is that.

MB: The piece of music which is very special for you is the quintet from Act 3 of *Die Meistersinger von Nürnberg*.

Die Meistersinger von Nürnberg, an opera by Richard Wagner

MB: This quintet is of real importance for you Keith. When did you first hear it?

Keith: I first heard it in Berlin in 1953 and at that point Wagnerian performances, with the exception of *Die Meistersinger*, were forbidden. So I was very interested. I knew little about it or what was going on but I do remember a long evening!

MB: How long was it?

Keith: Very long . . . about five hours . . . but the climax of the first scene in the third act had this wonderful music and the soprano singer was Elizabeth Grümmer who has always remained for me a model for this role. This quintet made an enormous impact upon me. It's the end of the private scenes in the opera. After this quintet it goes public. It brings together all the relationship strands which have gone before.

MB: We cannot appreciate the full text of the opera here but can you situate this quintet in the flow of the emotional plot for us?

Keith: An extremely complex set of relationships is investigated here in *Die Meistersinger*, played out against the backcloth of the competition for the best song, the prize song to be composed and performed in the town. There are intricacies about the rules and who is eligible but Walther is the hero who creates the winning song and Eva is his heroine. The complex relationships include the father–daughter dynamic. It's really interesting that that was a basic relationship for Verdi as well. The interest is not only with her real father Pogner, but also her 'other' father, if you like, Hans Sachs who is responsible for her re-birth into the world. The fact that they are sexually attracted to each other, and so on, has some very dark tones in the opera and one of the functions of the quintet I think is to resolve these difficult relationships as well as resolving the relationship between David, the very young apprentice, and his older lover Magdalene.

MB: We could say that we are looking at this opera with twenty-first century eyes. But do you think that Wagner would have been so overt in his writing and thinking of these dark tones?

Keith: Maybe unconsciously . . . I don't know . . . it's obviously there and it's there in the music because immediately before the quintet you have the enormous emotional outburst of Eva and the music begins to hint at this darkness.

MB: Eva is young and Hans Sachs is much older.

Keith: He has known her as a child . . . he tells her that he has seen her grow and now she has burst into full bloom. This is the moment of birth if you like . . . and this is played out against the prize song competition sung by her lover Walther. The prize song is considered as a baby which has to be christened . . . that is how the quintet is introduced . . . a new child has been born, the prize song, and we must officially christen it. And Walther if you like, has conceived this child in a dream, which is deeply interesting as well . . . pre-Freudian stuff . . . it's a wonderful act.

MB: Can you talk a bit about leitmotif Keith. It's an important musical device in Wagner . . . can you say a bit about its function and how it is used in this opera?

Keith: Its function is bound up with the psychological profundity of Wagner's work . . . he was not interested in the set arias and recitatives at this point. He moulded these together.

MB: And the leitmotif is what?

Keith: It is a melodic and/or rhythmic identification with a person or a mood or a philosophical idea. It can be identified with almost anything. Wagner's operas are also deeply interesting because the orchestra quite often expresses what cannot be said in the unfolding drama. This material is beyond language. There are some things that cannot be expressed in language.

MB: Or better not expressed in language?

Keith: Or better not expressed in language and we've just been talking about such content. This is another role of the leitmotif.

MB: That's fascinating.

Keith: And of course the leitmotif is infinitely flexible with key changes and parameters interweaving with one another. There's a comment I remember of a performance of *Die Meistersinger* overture. In the last couple of minutes of it there are many different tunes, leitmotifs, Beecham is conducting so you can hear each one! … but it's really the art of counterpoint, the interweaving, that is marvellous and *Die Meistersinger* is a joyous exploration of this.

MB: Opera in the hands of Wagner is a real music drama in that he wrote the words as well as the music. How do you understand Wagner's particular genius?

Keith: There is a new fashion now where people are really interested in the text of Wagner operas. But when I was younger the texts were either hopelessly obscure or considered too complex. Either way they were not considered very good. But things are changing in this respect … Wagner was interested in everything to do with opera, the visual, the stage production, the text and the music. There is a special opera house in Bayreuth built to accommodate all these aspects. I still hope to get there one day and perhaps really experience *Die Meistersinger von Nürnberg*.

MB: Thank you very much Keith.

References

1   Pater W (1873) *The Renaissance* (London 1873) essay on Giorgione.
2   Tippett M (1989) Art judgement and belief: towards the condition of music. In: P Abbs (ed.) *The Symbolic Order*. The Falmer Press, Sussex.

CHAPTER 5

Interview with William Angeloro

William Angelero is a producer/engineer working out of his studio, Handsome Llama Music Studios, in Frome, Somerset. In addition to this, he teaches music technology at Frome College as well as private tutelage. According to him his current musical obsessions are Norwegian jazz, Nick Drake, and the Master Musicians of Jajouka, He says that his wife still hates jazz!

Will's writing

My earliest memories of my *assigned* art form, music, are of sitting in my parents' apartment in Southern Brooklyn, New York, in the early seventies, listening to the sounds of Rossini's, *The William Tell Overture*. I was constantly exposed to a variety of different styles of music, moods or colours of sound (more on those terms later), such as salsa, classical, jazz, and the ever-present sixties and seventies rock and roll music. It was because of this saturation of sound at such a young, impressionable age that, maybe, I associate music with that feeling of awe and wonder of the world. A feeling we begin to lose, as we get older, as we assimilate all of our experiences into our personality, as we begin to understand the world.

Somewhere, imbedded in the very foundations of my mind, is the ability to hear music and use it to see everything around me, like I'm seeing it for the first time. No small joy for me, but a means to ecstasy. Perhaps listening to, say for instance, The Beatles *Abbey Road* album, or even James Brown, can take me to a time and place where my mind was open to the wonders of the world, gladly absorbing my surroundings and interpreting them as only a child may, without the distraction of the responsibilities that adulthood can bring, without the suppression of pure imagination.

Today, I consider myself an artist. I am a musician. I create art that inspires me. I create art that I hope will elicit the same response in others. What are these responses? I can only assume it is different for everybody, and I can only explain the responses to sound that are personal to me. For instance, since music has the power to bring me into a state of heightened awareness of the surrounding world (and the internal world), as explained earlier, I then can find myself hearing the music, almost visually. Sounds become colours, hues, smells and atmosphere. Louis Armstrong's *Hot Fives* is an almost brownish hue, a warm, crackling wood fire ambience. Anything from Stereolab is a kaleidoscope, leading my mind's eye on an almost, psychedelic journey. Beethoven allows me to imagine different worlds, or different versions of this world, depending on the piece.

As an almost antithesis to this, when there is *no* music around me, I compose a piece, or remember an appropriate piece to accompany what I am seeing or experiencing at that moment, in my mind. This is one of the deepest effects that art has had on me. My perception is always affected by sound and colour. Everything I see and feel and hear and taste, I, at once, associate with a sound and colour. The sound then brings about the appropriate openness and feelings of awe and inspiration, allowing me to live every moment like it's my first. So, you see, I can experience even the most mundane aspects of the daily grind, and use the experience to . . . weave a tapestry of sound, that serves a very practical purpose. It defines my existence.

This all may sound extreme, and almost, counterproductive to the practical world we live in, but it is not so. I believe, that in me at least, the honing of perception through art has allowed me to appreciate the beauty and the absurdity of life. It has enhanced a compassion for life that is sadly lacking in some aspects of modern society. It creates a spark of delight in performing the most menial of tasks, rather than hinder my ability to live in the 'real' world. An example of this may lie in my approach to my job. Say, for example, in my daily routine, I encounter a serious problem with the computer. Maybe this problem hinders a project I'm working on with an approaching deadline. Quite often, frustration and panic are the responses, followed by feelings of exasperation and confusion. And there is a deadline. But, as an artist, I'm trained to look at situations from all angles, to find alternative ways of viewing situations that may not necessarily be the first (or second, or third) way I would commonly approach it. Before any sense of defeat creeps in, I allow myself to step back from the problem, and in a sense, let it fix itself. The answer is somewhere; I just put myself in a position to be open to it. This type of mindset has forced me to think about situations and issues in an abstract way, and as a result, shaped my political, social and spiritual views.

They say art and music is dangerous, and it is, if you are the sort that needs to dominate the wills of others for your own gain, or the gains of your ideals. This is the reason that one of the first things Hitler *and* Stalin did when they came to power, was to regulate and control the arts. They knew that art *is* revolution. Not necessarily revolution in the 'armed uprising' sense, but a revolution of thought. It is said that art can change the world, and in this jaded, cynical world, most people laugh at the idea that anything can make a difference anymore. But the differences are small, and personal, and if music can have even the smallest, liberating effect on the mind, then it can move the populace into revolution; an intellectual and spiritual revolution.

Art and music means *that* much to me. It is, for me, a personal liberator. That is the job of the artist. To live the process and love the process of creating, and most of all, *be* the process of creation itself.

Conversation with Will

MB: Will, you write of music as your assigned art form, this almost feels as if there was no choice for you here, that you were born a musician?

Will: I was born an artist . . . music is what I use to express myself.

MB: You are 32 now . . . how did this artistic ability show itself in early years, at school for example?

Will: I used to play clarinet . . . this was my . . . first instrument. But from very early years with my parents it was the guitar. When I went to school I learned how to read music and from about the age of seven I played in an orchestra for about eight years. This was very frustrating in the early years because there was all this music and I couldn't really play it well enough on the instrument . . . very frustrating. When I went to college I decided I had to study music . . . so I began taking classes with the idea of getting a degree in music so I could teach. However, this changed when I went into strictly audio which is really the production end.

MB: That really began to interest you?

Will: I don't know when the technical side of studio work at college became so important, but the studio itself is an instrument.

MB: Yes . . . so not only could you play conventional musical instruments, you could use the technical musical equipment to make music too? Would that be right?

Will: Exactly . . . from that I went into production and became a producer. I produced other people's music at college. I used my ideas and my experience and knowledge to help other artists to bring their sound out. I influenced and pushed like a director would do in a movie, to get their product on tape and I've been doing that ever since.

MB: Right. You talk of your childhood in Southern Brooklyn New York and the varied music that you experienced. Can you say something about the people in your family who influenced you in music?

Will: My dad . . . there is a famous story that when I was brought back from hospital a few days old he put me next to the stereo so that I got used to it. I was always interested in what was being played. My dad said Jefferson Air Plane, the Southern California sixties hippie group, was the first 'rock and roll' I heard . . . I was three days old! So I was right in there. My dad had a strange esoteric taste in music. My mother loved swing . . . I had a little bit of both. But the second biggest influence was my father's brother, my uncle Al, who has to this day the largest record collection ever seen . . . tens of thousands. He introduced me to the 'blues' which I heard when I was six or seven. That absolutely changed me. He also introduced me to Spanish music, salsa, flamenco and African music.

MB: A huge variety of experience at home . . . so a very musical family in terms of listening?

Will: In terms of listening . . . I wouldn't be where I am without that.

MB: You write, Will, of music taking you to a different time and place . . . could you say more about this?

Will: There is the simple association of a smell or sound taking you back to a certain place . . . but for me I can hear a medieval madrigal and it will take me to that particular place in time. It's like an enhancement of where I am I think. Yea . . . I never feel I have to escape because I'm always looking around where I am. On the way here I was listening to Coltrane again and I can almost smell the smoke of a New York city bar. All music has that kind of texture for me.

MB: Mmn . . . you write of almost hearing music visually, what we would call synaesthesia . . . you don't say that about Beethoven though. Could you describe in colours or other senses any Beethoven piece that comes to mind?

Will: Yea Beethoven . . . the march from the *Ninth Symphony*. Somehow I always hear a version on the synthesiser which I heard when young. It has a kind of psychedelic quality, a sort of neon colouring. It was part of the film the *Clockwork Orange* and I snuck in to watch it . . . I was probably about eight or nine. But Beethoven is so vast . . . and its hard to be more specific. Synaesthesia is a difficult subject to talk about because it's so personal and might not be shared with others. As a composer . . . when I go outside and see how colours merge with one another I hear music. That's one of the best parts of being an artist. That particular combination of colours might be a pattern of sound or a progression of notes.

MB: It's as if they merge together in a new creative position for you . . . it's clear that music has a very practical purpose for you, as you say, in that it defines your existence. But tell me what your work was in New York when you finished at college?

Will: I made a conscious decision at 21 to try to make a living as a rock star . . . I put all my energy and money into playing in a particular band, composing the music, selling the image, doing the records and so on. After five or six years out of college I was doing clerk jobs in music shops, teaching on the side and a lot of boring day jobs to keep associated with music and musicians. The rest of the time in the band I was rehearsing, performing, practising, recording. That's all I did from age 21 to 28. I was writing my own stuff as well. Then more of the production side came in and I started working in recording studios to replace the day jobs and the more I got older the less I wanted to step up on stage . . . I wanted to get my ideas across and help other people get their ideas across and that's when I shifted into production and composing.

MB: And that has been successful?

Will: So far . . . but how do you measure success? Is it money? I haven't made so much money so far, but since I have stopped my mad run for rock stardom I think my music has gotten better. And really I have been having the grandest time being a musician.

MB: And in New York . . . You worked with young bands there?

Will: Yea . . . I was a part-time studio employee for seven years . . . I'm still really close to them. I engineered bands who just needed people to turn the knobs or I worked hand in hand with the composition, or the performance, or the production, or even the entire project. There are quite a few CDs out there with my name on them.

MB: Great, great! . . . so what do we call someone like you who does all these things?

Will: The producer I think . . . the producer oversees it all. But it involves many things. Right till the day I left New York last August there were three projects I was rushing to finish because I was moving to England and they came out fantastic. One was a 56-year-old woman who rediscovered her music career with a whole album based on housework. She had no band . . . just an acoustic guitar and her singing.

Will went on to describe the project which he worked on with her, how he built in a band for her with the computer, synthesiser and drum machines, and how they made a salsa record which is having moderate success right now. Her music is played in coffee houses, libraries and some pubs.

MB: Mmn . . . great . . . and where is your work here Will?

Will: Two years before I left the States I was strapped for money and right next to the studio I started working part-time in computers for an importing company, and when you have a steady income you sort of want to keep it, so I managed to stay with this guy and help him build up his business.

MB: What did he import?

Will: Oh . . . just jackets . . . ladies jackets from India. He sells them in the American market. It is a trading company with India. He started out as a long-haired back-packer in India, did a deal with this Indian couple to weave two jackets for them. He did a deal for some more and got all of this on a business footing when he got back to New York. They then started three little shops in New Delhi weaving these jackets. He still works with these same people now that he did 30 years ago. They are a little bit bigger now and are fantastically rich . . . one of them owns a house in St John's Wood. The employer is just a relaxed guy now.

MB: So you do some work for him?

Will: In the States I was in charge of computing his business. Next thing I know I was here to get married and working from here. As he says, 'Well what do you know why don't we try England and do some business there'. So we're still continuing in the States and giving it a shot here . . . which is great, so I can earn a bit of money while I set up my music business . . . which is my ultimate goal. I came to this trading business accidentally but it has been good.

MB: You sound as if you are very comfortable with it?

Will: I feel comfortable ... I've always been anti-sweat shop when it comes to workers. The first thing I did was look at this. Not only was it not a sweat shop business, but my friend has done a lot for these people and they've done a lot for us. It has worked both ways. He has had this relationship with them now for 30 years.

MB: You write about your music training framing your thinking to use alternative ways of viewing situations. What you do in your Indian project might be thought of as an alternative way of making money, a way where everybody wins or makes money?

Will: In the music business you have to learn how to take on yourself and delegate responsibility. I learned *that* in my import business. In my music work, which is the most important part of me, I have to make decisions that affect other people. That's why I say that music defines who I am and I couldn't live without it. Art has created my world. My music defines all. It is very serious. It is my method of achieving a sense of being.

MB: Yes ... that's right. Perhaps we can now have a look at *A Love Supreme* which is your chosen piece of music.

A Love Supreme – John Coltrane

In this jazz player's words, John Coltrane describes this piece as being in four parts – Acknowledgement, Resolution, Persuance and Psalm. In 1957 he describes what was for him a spiritual awakening and in 1964 the album, *Love Supreme*, was released. Before we talk about this spiritual awakening Will, can you say more about the roots of John Coltrane's spirituality?

Will: John Coltrane came from a Baptist upbringing I believe. His wife though was a devout Buddhist and her chant albums are considered the embodiment of John after he died. What so captures me about his music is probably the same thing that makes my wife Carolyn run screaming from the room. I've thought about this over and over. There are lots of pieces of music which bring out an extreme reaction in me. But there is something about his playing in general and his entire career which culminates and manifests itself in this piece especially the first part, Acknowledgement. I don't know clearly what he was trying to convey when he recorded it. He was so emotional and it was so powerful, so moving. It was like listening to a preacher ... as if someone was speaking 'in tongues'.

MB: Perhaps it was almost as if John Coltrane was talking to God?

Will: Right ... or ... a god ... that's the way I think. I don't necessarily believe in God but when I listen to that piece I feel I am being pushed to understand more than maybe is possible ... to understand about everything in some way. It is so beautiful and so harsh at the same time ... it is hard to explain.

MB: Can I ask whether you read the notes on it before you first heard it?

Will: Oh no! . . . I didn't realise who it was until I was about 12 years old. I didn't know why I liked it, the theme from the 'Acknowledgement'. Then came the question, What's going on? . . . It's him . . . it's his playing . . . very few players can keep up that intensity.

MB: Mmn . . . .

Will: The intensity was such that the people he was playing with have said that they would put their lives on the line to play that piece of music with him. That says how intense they all were and how much they believed in what they were trying to do.

MB: And what was it that they were trying to do?

Will: They were trying to elevate themselves . . . I think Coltrane was trying to save the world. I know he was! He felt that his music and music in general had . . . that essence that could bring out the best in people . . . and with the proper introduction at an early age and the proper appreciation, the proper exposure to music . . . people would think less about hitting each other for instance.

MB: I wonder perhaps if he was talking about the perception of some kind of order in life?

Will: I guess so . . . I think that's what his mission in life was . . . to bring out the best in people. I guess that's also what a lot of the great composers think . . . that they can add that little bit. In Southern California there is an actual Church of John Coltrane. It was felt that his dedication to love and peace was so profound that he should have a church dedicated to him.

MB: Yes . . . Mmn . . . . There is something else Will that I would like to explore with you. It's to do with the difference between classical music and jazz. There is a very significant difference in that classical music is usually written down and jazz relies on improvisation. There are a few exceptions like the cadenza in the classical concerto repertoire in which the soloist is invited to improvise without this part being written by the composer (although the composer's written cadenza is used by many soloists). What is it about the improvisation technique that so attracts you?

Will: Well . . . first off . . . jazz is written down in bare outline. I personally enjoy taking risks with performance in music . . . I like this space in music. When you are playing, the object of the playing is to forget you're doing it and then see what happens . . . it may be rather brilliant or it fails. Musicians have been trying to tap into this sort of depth of flow . . . is it God? . . . is it my muse? . . . is it the collective unconscious? I personally love getting myself into the position of either failing miserably in front of a crowd of people or producing the most beautiful sound experience ever and know that I'll never ever play that like that again.

MB: If you are playing in a group each needs to connect with the others. How do they do this?

Will: Yea . . . it's either eye contact with listening or listening alone. If you hear four people making a fantastic sound the energy builds up . . . it goes beyond the sound, it becomes the group itself and of course the audience comes in as well. It's no longer four individuals playing. It's a collective group experience and the audience joins in and encourages the players. This doesn't happen with classical music.

MB: Mmn . . . How far would you go along with the idea that immediacy, risk taking, aliveness, being present in and for the moment are phrases that one could use to describe a good jazz performance?

Will: Absolutely. The live show is what is important . . . records are less important . . . they are not the essence of the performance. The live communication between the players and the audience is the essence. But I know that I can never really be that high risk kind of jazz musician who just takes the heard phrase of sound and goes. I know that, that's why I do recording. I'm somewhere between. I use aspects of space and some improvisation.

MB: John Coltrane's work is inspired by his spiritual values . . . can you say something about your spiritual values?

Will: Very difficult . . . the only label I have been given is atheist, but that's not absolutely true. I believe in the energy around us, the connectedness of it all, and there may or may not be a higher power but if there is it is to do with connectedness. As a musician I want to tap into this spiritual energy. I don't know if there is a powerful mind at the top of this. I don't know and don't claim to know. When four guys are playing together, when they lock into this improvisational flow . . . where is it coming from? If you reach this state of mind . . . it's like a Buddhist meditation . . . can I not reach the heights of spirituality?

MB: There seems to be an intensity and gathering of feeling and sensation in the playing of music that is improvised. The emphasis in jazz seems to move into the performance and the performer rather than the music itself?

Will: Yes, I agree. With Beethoven the sound of notes on the page is the star of the show, whilst with jazz you've got to hear and preferably *see* the performer play. The big stars could play nursery rhymes and people would flock to hear them. So it's not what he's playing, it's how he's playing it . . . with an orchestra you firstly want to hear what they're playing.

MB: I think we may be talking about emphasis. In a symphony the focus is on the music. There is no soloist. In the jazz performance the focus is on the performer playing the music, whilst in a classical concerto the soloist and the music are attended to almost equally and this is nearer the experience of the personal performer in jazz.

Will: In jazz the experience of listening to the performer and the immediacy and risk of their live performance is what a good concert is about.

MB: Whilst we might say that the classical concert is an interpretation of the creativity of the composer distilled into music on the page?

Will: Yes, I absolutely agree. What you have just said would in no way apply to a jazz concert. Music which is written down and worked over has a certain quality about it that improvisation doesn't have and improvisation has a quality about it that classical music doesn't have. As a pop composer with a classical background I feel I couldn't put out a recording without working it over there and then. Also there is no way I could make a recording that's devoid of improvisation. I guess I've got a foot in both worlds.

MB: How comfortable is that Will?

Will: For me it's perfect!

MB: Thank you Will.

Will then played one of his recorded compositions for me full of layering of sound. It would be played in coffee shops or college campuses. As he said, 'It unfolded to take us somewhere'. As it unfolded it became an improvised meeting of different styles.

CHAPTER 6

Interview with Maggie Senior

Maggie Senior is a psychotherapist and tutor in psychotherapy living in Nottingham. She has an interest in the role of creativity and personal narrative in psychotherapy.

Maggie's use of the term 'replacement baby' needs some explanation. A replacement baby is known in the field of psychotherapy as an infant born within a year of the death of a child who would have been a year-old brother or sister. The earlier child would perhaps have been a still birth or would have died within a few weeks of being born. A replacement baby therefore, in this instance Maggie, is understood as being born into a grief-stricken family. Any such family may move too quickly in trying to welcome the new child while still suffering greatly from the loss of the earlier one.

Maggie's writing

I am a replacement baby who grew up with quite musical parents; my mother sang, loved poetry and literature and my father played the piano well. His passion was Beethoven, whose sonatas he played endlessly. Through music they communicated their grief for their dead daughter who died a year before I was born. Through music and words my father communicated his grief and the terror of his war experiences, shooting Germans and opening up the concentration camps whose smell he remembered until his death.

I learned to access my own emotions through music. I had to cut so much off in me when I was a child, because their (my parents') grief, terror and anger was so great. But music (choral singing mainly when I was younger) helped me gain a sense of my own history, a sense of who I am in the world, a sense of my own emotionality, a sense of passion and love and fun. There was fun as well in our household; sometimes my Dad and I would play duets, or my mum would sing and read poetry. I was brought up on AA Milne and RL Stevenson and still love the sound and rhythms of words as well as the sound and rhythm of music.

I was a very vigilant child and noted both the sounds and emphases of my parents' expression, as well as the spaces in between the sounds. This 'musical ear' served me well as a therapist noting the pace and rhythms of a client's words, what they say, don't say and what my own tune is – whether I felt harmonised, or not, for example. The other thing about music is that I can get caught up in something much greater than me. Not only does it define me individually, I can lose that and be caught up collectively, so to speak.

Perhaps I should also stress that I have a very catholic musical taste. I listen to anything and everything, from Jimmy Hendrix to Shamanic chanting, from Sibelius to Bach. About the only thing I have a bit of difficulty with is country and western, mainly because I associate it with the sentimentality of the Deep South and racism.

Let me finish from Act 3, Scene 2 of *The Tempest.* Caliban speaks:

> Be not afeard. The isle is full of noises,
> Sounds, and sweet airs, that give delight, and hurt not.
> Sometimes a thousand twangling instruments
> Will hum about my ears; and sometime voices,
> That, if I then had wak'd after long sleep,
> Will make me sleep again; and then in dreaming,
> The clouds methought would open and show riches
> Ready to drop upon me, that, when I waked
> I cried to dream again.

And finally, Lorenzo from *The Merchant of Venice*, Act 5, Scene 1:

> The man that hath no music in himself
> Nor is not mov'd with concord of sweet sounds
> Is fit for treasons, stratagems and spoils;
> The motions of his spirit are dull as night,
> And his affections dark as Erebus,
> Let no such man be trusted.

Conversation with Maggie

MB: Maggie, you talk of being a replacement baby and we understand something of what this might have meant for you being born into such a grieving family context. You talk about your parents' grieving relationship with each other but you don't talk much about your relationship with them.

Maggie: Yes, that's right . . . that's left me wondering about what kind of relationship I did have with them. I was put into a nursery at the age of two and was told endlessly by my mum what a lucky little girl I was. There was music there at the nursery, and that was good. My principle relationship was with my grannie, my father's mother. My dad was out at work a lot and grannie was my mainstay. My recollection of my mum was sort of utilitarian . . . bathing me, dressing me, etc.

MB: Were there any brothers or sisters?

Maggie: No . . . I was quite an isolated child.

MB: You talk of access to your emotions through music, but also somehow that you had to cut off this access?

Maggie: Yes, it was as if their joint grief blotted out my confusion and isolation. It was bigger than me and my needs . . . I became very introverted but I had an outward sense of 'okayness' . . . I defined myself as an extrovert/introvert. Music became a vehicle for me in which to be and also an invasion of me . . . it was a vehicle to carry emotion for me and I could seek to understand it there. But I would also have to turn it off . . . not allow it inside my body . . . it was too much! The music I listen to now and in recent years, and which I most enjoy, has this dialogue about it; duets or quartets. I have been listening to Rachmaninov's *Cello Sonata*, cello and piano dialoguing together with the cello providing the ground and the piano decorating on top . . . a 'give and take' quite different from the dialogue between my parents which was clashing and dissonant.

MB: I wonder if this musical dialogue is also a different experience from the dialogue between your parents in that you are allowed into this dialogue in music?

Maggie: Yes, I am allowed into it. I belong in this musical dialogue. This feeling of being included is very important for me.

Maggie goes on to talk about her isolation at home and her feelings of not being included. Choral singing came to her rescue in that it allowed her to transcend her own individuality and experience something greater, holding and perhaps healing.

MB: It seems that music was a kind of therapeutic frame for you. We talk about a therapeutic frame in your professional life as a psychotherapist. I wonder if it is too much to say that music attuned you to the dynamic textures and the rhythms and pace of your therapeutic practice?

Maggie: Yes, I think it really did. It helped me to attune myself to the clients and 'their music'.

Maggie went on to parallel the therapeutic conversational aspects of rhythms and silences with rhythms and silences in music and the subtle nuances of tone of voice in the client's narrative with timbre of sound and the concept of musical flow. She continued . . .

Maggie: The more we meet with a client the more we begin to hear these many subtle aspects of her narrative, for example, the spaces between words which are part of her music. And it takes a while to tune into this and really to hear *how* she expresses herself; who she is.

MB: Her inner music?

Maggie: Yes, and the different nuances of this, how the flow of her narrative might change suddenly as a rhythm or a key in music changes, and what this might be about for her.

MB: Changing key here, as it were ... you talk about the experience of music sometimes, as if it feels like being caught up in something greater than you ... being caught up collectively in a larger experience. Can you say a bit more about this?

Maggie: I'll try ... I go to an image, not about music but an image about transcending pain. I used to ski a lot. When I was feeling desperate in my marriage I remember looking out on the Bella Vada ski run, the beautiful way, and it is a tough bloody run! I had done this run earlier in the day and was thrilled about this ... I woke up in the middle of the night, looked out and there was a huge moon, the colour of deep brass, and the dark sky was a colour of deep, deep lapis. During the darkest moments of my marriage I woke up on one occasion and the bedroom was illuminated by this vision of light. The experience was outside me, inside me, it was me ... and I just sat in awe. It was as if the bedroom was full of light and mountain and so was I. I thought what's this all about? And a tremendous peace came over me.

MB: So there is something greater?

Maggie: Yes ... something greater than my pain, and this is also what music gives me. The being caught up by it and the thought that this music is going to be heard over succeeding generations. This music will play on even though it is not sounding to me at this moment. It still plays, it's still there.

MB: It's still sounding somewhere in the world?

Maggie: Yes, somewhere. This is the spiritual aspect of it. I'm not talking about religion here. I am talking about spirit.

MB: At this point, can you say something about your Catholic taste in music; your broad taste in music?

Maggie: The only things I have real trouble with in this area are country and western singing and the thump thump noise which usually is heard from a passing car radio. I will listen to almost anything but this stuff I can't abide. This whole context of thump thump sounds is without grace.

MB: But the person experiencing these thump thump sounds would claim to be listening to music. So what makes what we call music different from this?

Maggie: The way this thump thump sound is produced is mechanical, predictable and it rules the individual. If you take the score of a Mozart piano concerto, although the notation is there, fixed on paper, the sounds produced by the pianists would be different in each performance. There is room for a different kind of engagement each time; different forms of intimacy.

MB: Are you saying that in the thump thump sounds there is no response other than feeling bludgeoned?

Maggie: Yes, it feels like being bludgeoned, overwhelmed and having my individuality crushed.

MB: Almost as if you really become obliterated by this experience. There is no reverie, you don't have space to think, to dream?

Maggie: There is no dream, no reverie, no delicacy. It feels like a holocaust . . .

MB: A dead quality about it? I wonder if you include 'heavy metal' here?

Maggie: Oh! No . . . I love heavy metal . . . it's the modern computerised stuff, because it's without soul. It's mechanised. Jimmy Hendrix tuning his guitar strings I love . . . *Purple Haze* . . . any day . . . love it . . . atonal music? . . . I also love Messiaen's work. Jazz I love, trad, and modern . . . music from the East, Gamelan, Indian music. The country and western I can't take because it's without soul. It doesn't include you . . . it assaults you.

MB: This sounds an almost frightening experience that *you* know about from somewhere?

Maggie: I think that I took in a lot of my parents' fears. They were very frightened people . . . they were afraid I would die. Also my father had gone through the war and he had experienced the terror of the concentration camps . . . these were people who were traumatised and he was too . . . so there is something about terror and fear being a very bodily experience and music soothes that . . . music gets into the body and heals it I think.

MB: Yes . . . even though music is thought to be the most abstract of the arts, as you say, it gets inside you . . . perhaps more powerfully than the other arts? . . . I may be pushing this a bit.

Maggie: My sense is that music is particularly powerful here and does get into the middle part of the brain; into the limbic system, not necessarily the higher functions of thought.

MB: There is some experimental work going on involving playing Mozart to children in the classroom. They are said to be able to think better. This may be about balance and the shaping of sounds and phrasing in Mozart . . . and the inevitability of the next note?

Maggie: It's containing.

MB: Yes, a holding which is ordered but not rigid?

Maggie: Yes, yes and cows enjoyed being milked better too!

MB: Having claimed that appreciation of music such as a Mozart piano concerto brings out the spiritual in humankind, I wonder if you could say more about this higher quality?

Maggie: In the thump thump sounds there is no space for dialogue anywhere in the experience. Engagement with an – 'other' – is missing. Real music is about an intimate dialogue. Martin Buber[1] writes on the experience of I–Thou and I–It. Music for me is about I–Thou. The thump thump experience is I–It, an object that is crushed, dehumanised. When I listen to Mozart, I am included in a mutual exchange, between me and the humanity of which the music speaks. I am in it . . . held within a sanctuary . . . a sanctity . . . a safe place, a holy place . . . yes!

MB: Is there a particular piece of music which articulates . . . who you are Maggie?

Maggie: Yes . . . it would have to be one of Beethoven's last string quartets . . . probably the A minor, and the movement that I know as the 'Holy Thanksgiving'.

MB: Perhaps we could talk a bit about this piece?

Maggie: Yes I'd like to do that because at an emotional level it links with my Dad, and also Beethoven himself seems very much to remind me of my father.

We then talked about how this piece was written when Beethoven was recovering from serious illness and also completely deaf. Both his illness and his inability to hear would have brought about a deep sense of isolation in him. Maggie then continued to reflect upon isolation.

Maggie: In many ways I had an isolated and isolating childhood and being an only child . . . and in some ways . . . my parents sealed off . . . sealed off from me emotionally . . . this music articulated this isolating experience . . . and therefore connects with me when I hear it. But it doesn't just do that . . . it has a weight, a gravitas, about it in its articulation. But it isn't just the story of Beethoven's sadness and his grief nor an exploration of these aspects . . . it lifts and enhances and transcends and articulates that which goes beyond this isolating experience.

MB: Mmn . . . and this for you . . . would be the spiritual?

Maggie: Yes . . . it is . . . I think . . . the spiritual dimension of the music . . . a holy place . . . I don't quite know what more to say about the spiritual.

After a while Maggie went on to consider this safe holding place as a sanctuary in which she feels met, recognised, affirmed and added to in some way.

MB: You say you are somehow made more you?

Maggie: Made more me . . . mmn . . . because in isolation we can split off . . . we can become numb . . . and desensitise. But this music brings back to me something . . . that is not split off . . . that is welcomed, welcoming. I am included in the experience and I grow from it. The Beethoven experience does not detract, does not take away from.

MB: But the experience of the concentration camp did take away from your father. I wonder what you think his experience of Beethoven would have meant for him after that awful time?

Maggie: I think he felt very conflicted because he loved Beethoven before he went to Germany and then the concentration camp was his real German experience.

MB: So he is met with something that is alien to what he knows of Beethoven as a German from the piano sonatas?

Maggie: Yes . . . Yes.

MB: He doesn't know what to do with this?

Maggie: He doesn't know what to do with this. How can this be?

MB: But he continues to listen to Beethoven?

Maggie: Yes, he continues to listen to Beethoven and play it . . . play it for hours.

MB: There *is* something there, something more?

Maggie: I know it is more than me. It also enhances me . . . I grow from it. It is more, goes beyond me, goes beyond me and the purely personal.

MB: And by that, you don't mean the impersonal?

Maggie: No, the interpersonal, the collective, us, and perhaps the transpersonal, goes beyond the individual, even, that is me, that was my father. The experience of the concentration camps was a collective insanity, a madness, a taking away from . . . a meaninglessness, so this, through Beethoven's music goes into a collective positive experience as the sound goes beyond this sound held in this moment of time. Generation after generation has heard this, been given to and enhanced by this.

   We go on to reflect on Beethoven's personal struggle with deafness and how he had to be turned around at the end of the first performance of his *Ninth Symphony* so that he could *see* the applause because he could not hear it.

Maggie: I can only speculate what he must have felt, moved to tears . . . to joy . . . affirmed . . . made human. Beethoven's sense of empty isolation reminds me of the experience of the small baby. A baby who is not recognised by his or her mother in a loving look, or in a loving sound . . . isn't filled up . . . isn't affirmed. . . . a shell.

MB: And it needs to be met and filled somewhere?

Maggie: Yes, that's right.

MB: You could say that deafness pushed Beethoven into this kind of place?

Maggie: Yes.

MB: So . . . it is in people . . . the 'I–thou' experience that Martin Buber[1] talks about. It is in connection and communication with people that we . . .

Maggie: It is in the loving affirming look of mother to child that we are first affirmed, that we begin to find our spirituality, our connectedness and communication, our spiritual nature . . . it's also like Moses coming down from the mountain top where he has been in spiritual isolation. He comes back with his thoughts and greets the tribe. It is interconnectedness.

MB: Yes, like Beethoven, as he was turned round.

Maggie: With his tablets or his music . . . this is it.

MB: I've found it . . . it's been there all the time. It's in the interconnectedness . . . it's in the engagement.

Maggie: In the giving to . . .

MB: Well . . . we're near to the word love.

Maggie: Yes.

MB: Do you want to take this a bit further?

Maggie (laughter): Well, I'm not ever so good at Greek but it's more that Eros and Agape. It is about compassion . . . it's not eroticism . . . that may be an expression of it. But it is about compassion.

MB: Feeling with . . .

Maggie: Com . . . yes, with . . . the passion of life.

MB: Which we have to be alongside, and 'with'.

Maggie: And that was what was lacking in the holocaust experience . . . there was no feeling 'with'.

MB: That's right . . . a death dealing experience.

Maggie: A death experience also, literally and psychically seen and experienced by my father.

MB: Of course. For Beethoven . . . for your father and somewhere for you?

Maggie: Mmn . . . I have spoken about my connectedness with my father through music. I would sit at his piano stool and listen to the sounds of the piano . . . a bit like Beethoven would have to when he was playing. Because I was little I would sit underneath and listen to the sounds of the piano with my ear against it.

MB: As if you were held in the music in the presence of your father?

Maggie: Yes, held by it. Yes, given to and communicated with. I can still feel this ear against the piano you know . . . and it would echo in my head . . . it still echoes in my head.

MB: Still echoes?

Maggie: I listen to it over and over. I listen to music now over and over again and carry it in my head. I'm sure I did that as a child.

Maggie and I move on to talking more specifically about the Holy Hymn of Thanksgiving from the Beethoven *String Quartet in A minor*.

Beethoven *String Quartet opus 132 in A minor*, the third movement Molto Adagio – Holy Hymn of Thanksgiving

This third movement of the Beethoven *String Quartet in A minor* has a particular form ABABA which is in itself a musical device. The A section is an introduction of the material, the B section is a complete contrast. The A section returns and we then have a repeat of the B section and then the final A section. I asked Maggie if she might like to say something about the flow from one state to the other.

Maggie: In the beginning in those long drawn-out chords there is a sense of isolation in the first A section. Then the B section has more energy. There is a lift to it.

MB: A stately dance?

Maggie: Yes. It is a dance but not a hugely energetic dance. Well, it's almost like a slow gavotte.

MB: Yes, that in and from this isolation we can move . . .

Maggie: Move to dance . . . yes.

Maggie goes on to talk of the problems of sitting still when listening to music. She feels she wants to go with the music, she wants to dance, and to sit rigidly listening to music in a concert hall is alien to her. In the B section of this piece, however, she wants to dance but in a slightly halting way.

Maggie: I ask myself, 'What does this mean in my body?' . . . it's not a triumphant dance . . . I almost feel as if . . . I'm slightly lame in some kind of way . . . slightly lame . . . wounded.

MB: Not the free exhuberant dance of his *Seventh Symphony*?

Maggie: Absolutely not that . . . I'm lame . . . but I can still dance.

We talk further about the return of the long drawn-out chords of the A section, reminding the listener of the isolation and the nature of illness, the nature of pain and grief. The 'holding on' feeling as it were, but then the B section returns for a second time and everything changes. We know that Beethoven has lightness and humanity because we have heard his dance, his lameness in the first B section. But this time, there is a different quality about this return of the B section.

Maggie: It is still a lame dance yes, but the second time around of this B section we hear that the dance is not crippling. It seems to be more forceful . . . it's not aggressive . . . more defined somehow . . . more definite . . . more self-assured.

MB: I'm a lame person? . . . almost a shaking of the fist?

Maggie: Yes It's more vigorous . . . more human. I am not going to be crushed by this experience.

MB: Beethoven moves in his lameness.

Maggie: And we want to move with it.

MB: So we feel connected up, not only listening *to* the flow of distant humanity in the A section, as if the long drawn-out chords are a disembodied flow. We are now connected up with the body . . . we are not split off from the body.

Maggie: We are most aware of this sense of connectedness with the body when we return to the last A section, the final section, and we hear this familiar music from a different place . . . from a more human place and we reflect again . . . it seems to contain so much of everything that has gone before. It is an inclusive statement over a period of time, which holds the whole piece together.

MB: It would seem that the whole movement could be described in these terms. We could say that the first A statement, the opening long drawn-out chords is about humanity's isolation. Then there is the first experience of the B section telling the world of Beethoven's humanity, the bodily experience. The A section returns with the reflective chords and then we hear the B section for a second time almost saying, perhaps, 'I'm still here – and it doesn't get any better'.

Maggie: "But I'm still here" . . . and then the last A section . . . it's inclusive and affirming! It includes elements of both suffering humanity and peace. It is not either/or which we have been presented with earlier. It is both/and . . . therefore . . . "This is me. Yes".

MB: "Can you hear me?"

Maggie: Mmn . . . and his experience was that he was heard . . . his quartets were heard . . . he was met . . . and he is still being met . . . and that was probably enough . . . ?

MB: Of course. Thank you very much Maggie.

References

Buber M (1971) *I and Thou*. Simon and Schuster, New York and London.

CHAPTER 7

Interviews with Safiya Mohammad; Wajiha Mohammad and Roopa Nair

Safiya Mohammad 26, was born and educated in India. She is housewife to Fahim Mohammad 34, and lives with her mother-in-law, in Northampton. Safiya is happily occupied in bringing up her little two-year-old boy, Faiz.

Wajiha Mohammad 47, was born and educated in London. She was married and lived in India for ten years. She now lives with her 11-year-old daughter Adeeba, in Northampton. Wajiha is Course Director for Black and Asian Studies at Leicester University (Northampton Centre) and Course Leader of counselling courses at Northampton College. Wajiha's brother Fahim is married to Safiya.

When Roopa Nair did her interview for this book she lived and worked in Derby. During the writing of the book she married Som Kumar and has now moved to live in India.

The experience of music from a different culture

This chapter is arranged differently from the others. I originally wanted to explore the experience and meaning of Indian music for an individual listener, only to find out that I had taken on an enormous task. Who could I ask about this experience of listening to Indian music? Would it be a Hindu or a Muslim listener or a member of one of the many other different religious ways of being in this complex culture which is India.

The cultural and religious differences in this large sub-continent are so numerous that no one view of music in particular would be truly representative of Indian music. I could of course have concentrated on the intricacies of Indian music itself and how these are rooted in cultural and religious differences within

India, but this book is not the place for this kind of study. I decided therefore to concentrate on in-depth conversations with individual listeners from the Muslim and the Hindu faiths. However, I discovered an even greater difficulty here which I had not foreseen.

In my early attempts at these interviews I was feeling increasingly lost. I then realised that I was asking questions from a Western perception of self and self-in-relation which is entirely different from the Indian sense of self-in-community. When I tried asking questions requiring an individual personal response there was a constant slippage in the answers from an individual response into a community response. For example, if I asked 'What do you feel about such and such?', the answer might be 'In India we do this . . .' or 'We experience music . . .'. This is an exaggeration to make a point. But as the questions became more meaningful and more in-depth, this kind of slippage became more frequent. It began to feel impossible.

It then became apparent to me that I was not hearing the complexity of the Indian identity which is *community* first and then *self* which is not the usual Western frame of interpersonal engagement, except perhaps, for some rural, church and religious communities where their very survival depends on communal living. Realising the source of my difficulty I decided to modify my interview so as not to trample on a sense of self-in-community of which I knew very little.

Three Indian women then generously agreed to be interviewed. They are each in the process of negotiating who they are as developing persons in this very different Western culture of England and the interviews seemed to centre on this aspect. As we began to talk I quickly realised for the first time something of the depth of the kind of struggle each was engaged in, in her own way. They all have deep roots in India through the extended family and their specific community and they must retain this personal/community integrity at the same time as having to respond appropriately to the individualistic world outside this community in this Western society. They are therefore required to balance constantly the heavy weight of tension between the individual Western sense of selfhood, which they experience in any communication they have with a Westerner, with the equally powerful sense of self-in-community in which each has been brought up.

They are all at different stages and with different challenges in their journey of East/West integration. Because of this the interviews are shorter, but what each shows us is how difficult this journey has been and still is. I am deeply grateful to Safiya Mohammad, her sister-in-law – Wajiha Mohammad – who helped out during the interview, and Roopa Nair for allowing me to share something of their chosen pathways.

Safiya's writing

When I listen to music both my thoughts and feelings are ignited. Memories return depending on the type of music. Slow-paced music relaxes me and fast-paced music makes me feel excited and happy. I'm usually made happy by music. However, my initial mood is always intensified. If I'm already feeling happy, then music makes me feel happier. If I'm feeling sad, then the music may sadden my mood further.

If I particularly like a piece of music, I'm very aware of the musical flow. I find myself concentrating and listening to the plot very carefully. I'm aware of all the high notes and the crescendo of the musical piece. All my thoughts and feelings are intensified.

My strongest memory is that of my father listening to his tapes of Indian songs. His favourites were from the Indian films called *Umrao Jaan* and *Nikaah*. This type of music is called 'ghazals', i.e. the music and lyrics are based on poetry. I remember I was five years old at the time. I also remember the huge loud speakers on the streets and shops of our village playing Indian film music. The temples also had religious music and songs playing in the background. The temple music all sounded similar to me as I used to walk past. I can remember the closeness I shared as I walked by with my sisters, friends and cousins. They were very happy and carefree times.

I experienced a very normal childhood, in fact I would say that I remained emotionally the same until I was 17 years old!! Then I became more responsible because of my college studies, my home life (which included entertaining family and friends), learning to sew, to do embroidery and cook. I remember doing all these with my mother, sisters and friends. Also, my elder sisters were in the process of getting married. This brought about all the expectations and excitement of new members being added to our family. I was very keen in wanting to get to know both my new brother-in-laws.

I also remember that behind my house was a 'talkie' cinema and they always played the same song over and over again for years – *Meri Desh Ki Dharti* (The soil of my homeland). This was played at least seven or eight times a day. As this is a very patriotic song I have always linked it to my life, even to this day. Now, even though I live in England, whenever I hear this song, I'm transported back to my home village of Lanji in central India. All my senses are affected: the warmth of the Indian weather, my family and friends; the smell and taste of the foods; the beautiful green fields and farms. The depth of the greenery and the colours are most memorable.

Words such as 'joy' and 'happiness' spring to mind of these times. I remember being with my family the most. I was closest to my sister Rafia and my mother. I remember my childish fights and arguments with my youngest sister Sanju. It was when I turned about 16 or 17 that I first remember getting really close to my elder brother Shakeel. It was talking about music that brought us together. He has always loved listening to Indian film songs too. He was the most interested in and most knowledgeable of music at that time. He could also afford to buy his own cassettes at the time too. I remember becoming closer to him at this stage of my life.

I have always loved fast-paced music. Now I'm drawn to slow-paced and classical styles of music. I have always loved the sound of the flute. There is one particular piece of music in the Indian film *Hero* of the early 1980s that I have loved from the first time I heard it. This particular tune is very beautiful and touches my heart in an unexplainable way. I just concentrate on the tune, the melody and nothing else. My mind actually becomes empty to anything else around me. I become totally absorbed in the melody. It is very beautiful and haunting. The composer and player of this piece is Pundit Hari Prasad Chaurasia, a very eminent and respected musician in India.

Slow classical music by Nusrat Fateh Ali Khan (the famous Pakistan 'Quwalli' singer) has always been another important influence in my taste and experience of music. His music has made me a better listener and given me more appreciation of quality music. His work affects me emotionally, by making me sensitive to other people's feelings, their pain, separation and losses. Yet, at the same time it highlights how lucky I am in my very content lifestyle. Thank God my life is routine and on the same level always. I have not experienced the highs and lows life offers some other people. Thankfully I'm truly content and blessed.

Now marriage to Fahim and becoming a mother to a very energetic little boy of two, Faiz, has lessened the time I can spend listening to music. Although music is always playing in the background on the TV (the Indian music channel B4U) or on the radio, there are far fewer times when I'm truly drawn to a particular piece of music. This may be due to my total concentration of caring for my baby. Yet, now it is the music or tunes my son likes that I'm drawn too. The recent Indian film *Ghadar* has an old-fashioned style of music, based on Indian folk music. It is this music my son absolutely loves. He stops doing whatever he is doing and just listens to this music when it comes on the TV or radio. I'm now drawn to this piece of music as it brings so much happiness to my son. I feel so proud and happy when Faiz 'hums' to this music, even though he cannot speak words yet!!

Since becoming a mother my responsibility and concentration are on looking after Faiz. I don't buy as many music cassettes or CDs as before. However, the TV and radio are always playing Indian song music in the background. I don't specifically sit down and listen to music anymore as I don't have the time now. But I'm still aware of it in the background, especially through my son's reactions to music. I'm not very keen on current Western music trends, as it is too loud and the lyrics are difficult to understand or appreciate.

Without music life would be empty, silent and quiet. I will always appreciate music in my life. I'm most drawn to the lyrics in music. This along with good quality music and melody, either sad or happy, makes what I feel good music is all about.

Conversation with Safiya, assisted by Wajiha

MB: Music is very important for you Safiya and you remember hearing tapes of Indian songs when you were five. Where was your home and who was there with you?

Safiya: My home was in a small village, Lanji, in central India and I lived there with my mum, dad, three sisters and my brother.

MB: You write of your father seeing the films in the 'talkie' cinema behind the house. Did you see any of these when you were young?

Safiya: Yes I did see some of them with my dad when I was five or six.

MB: You write of a kind of music in the films called ghazals. Can you say a bit more about this kind of music?

Safiya: It is very slow and the lyrics are very meaningful.

MB: What are they about Safiya?

Safiya: They are romantic songs for lovers.

MB: You say that you remember the huge loud speakers in your village playing film music and also the temple music at the same time . . . it all sounds a bit noisy. What about silence . . . was there much silence?

Safiya: The music was coming from far away so it was not too noisy.

MB: So it was background music in the distance . . . what did you feel about this?

Safiya: You got used to it . . . it was part of your life growing up and you got used to it.

MB: Tell me a bit more about the temple music which all sounded the same?

Safiya: Some of the temple singing is based on the film music.

At this point Wajiha, Safiya's sister-in-law helped out in my confusion. It seems that the temple plays film music to cater for the younger generation . . . pop music too!!

MB: You talk about your family and friends, Safiya, and it sounds as if there was always someone there and you were never lonely.

Safiya: Yes . . . this was a good feeling. My cousins and my uncle lived nearby and used to visit every day. My sisters were there also and their friends who were neighbours. Neighbours are very friendly in India. My father is a doctor and patients come to the house . . . they used to come in and talk with my mum . . . so there were people coming and going all, the time.

MB: Now that's very interesting . . . the patients would come and talk with your mum and be friendly with everybody round about . . . that's very different in this country when a patient goes to the doctor.

Safiya: Yes . . . very very different.

MB: It would be the practice here that if you had to go to the doctor in his house everyone would have to keep out of the way. That's not the way in India?

Safiya: People would come and see my dad, get a prescription and then go and see my mum and have a cup of tea . . . so the whole day there would be people coming and going.

MB: I am fascinated by this Safiya. So what about what we call over here . . . patient confidentiality. This means that what is said to the doctor never goes anywhere else. How does that work in the circumstances you describe?

Safiya: It depends on the doctor . . . yes, it depends on the doctor.

Wajiha came to the rescue by saying that if it was a serious matter and the patient wanted confidentiality then that is respected. But, generally, if the doctor's family is around, the position is that the family is part of the practice and flexibility in confidentiality is accepted.

MB: You went to college at 17 Safiya. What did you study there?

Safiya: I studied and have a BSc in mathematics, physics and chemistry.

MB: And what did you want to do with this degree?

Safiya: I always wanted to be a housewife . . . (I must have had a quizzical expression on my face because Safiya continued) . . . honestly . . . because if you go to work in India, when you come home you still have to do everything. But I will work here when I have more time . . . when my son is older.

MB: How would you have more time here?

Safiya: Life is easier here . . . there are washing machines, floor cleaning machines, dishwashers. Here for instance for cooking there are mixers and grinders, but in many rural areas of India all of this has to be done by hand and there are a lot of visitors all the time who eat with us . . . open house.

MB: This sounds very time-consuming too. I do understand that you can't do that and an outside job as well. It's just not possible. You write about your sister getting married. Can you tell me about getting married in this part of India?

At her sister's wedding Safiya described the process of getting married in the Muslim tradition as a simple ceremony in the presence of the Maulana, the priest, and 300 people! The Maulana asks the bridegroom and bride three times if they want to marry. Each has to answer in turn, 'Yes . . . yes . . . yes'. There is a prayer to God to wish them a happy marriage and it is over. I asked Safiya if this was an arranged marriage.

Safiya: Yes . . . I myself have always wanted an arranged marriage. In my own marriage I fell in love with my husband after we were married.

MB: That is lovely Safiya . . . but I must say I am fascinated at the 300 people attending your sister's wedding . . . what happens as a celebration?

Safiya: There is a feast.

MB (with some incredulity): There is a feast for 300 people? . . . and who would pay for all of this?

Safiya: In my own marriage my father paid for this.

Wajiha then explained that there would be a minimum of 300 guests and often the numbers would go as high as 1000.

MB: And tell me about the music at this celebration.

Safiya: There is no music at the ceremony . . . there are readings from the Holy Book – the Qur'an.

Wajiha added that although there is no music at the ceremony, there may be music at the party a few days later, in the background. After the marriage has been consummated there is another feast and the bridegroom's father pays for this feast. But because Safiya's father is very religious there was no music at her wedding. Interestingly, Safiya's father loves music but it would not be played at such a formal occasion. There are lots of families who don't have music at weddings. It is part of Islamic cultural tradition that there is no music. But in modern Islamic culture it is beginning to be heard. The Qur'an traditionally is the music of Islam. It has beautiful rhythm and when people hear it they are emotionally moved.

MB: So the music is in the words?

Wajiha: Islam teaches that the rhythm is in the words of God and it is absolutely beautiful. I myself have witnessed this . . . when we pray we can feel it. Listening to music itself is very un-Islamic because it is said to lead you towards the devil. Sounds on musical instruments are said to take you away, away from the divine . . . from the Book . . . music can lead you into that which is enthralling . . . it can lead you to the passions and to dream about physical love. So, in Islam you fall in love after the wedding ceremony with the Qur'an as the gateway. You don't have boyfriend and girlfriend relationships, what in the West used to be called courting, and music can awaken these kinds of passions before marriage and therefore is forbidden.

MB: Thank you Wajiha. There is a piece of music you talk about Safiya *Meri Desh Ki Dharti* (The soil of my homeland) and it reminds you of your home in India. I wonder what you feel when you hear this song now living in England?

Safiya: When I hear this song it takes me back to my village, my soul goes to my village and I feel upset because I'm not there.

MB: In this country we call this homesickness and this feels very sad for you. This is also very understandable in that the weather is so awful and the customs are so very different. However, your chosen music is *Piya re* sung by the Quwalli singer Nusrat Fateh Ali Khan and is about the pain of separation and loss. Are you able to say more about this Safiya?

Piya re

My love (Piya re)
Without you my mind and heart are restless.
Your eyes have caught me under their magic.
Without you I am restless. My heart beats in distress when I'm without you.
The flute plays its tune for you to listen to me.
Without you there is no meaning for me.
My love, my love, my love.
Your eyes have caught me under their magic. Without you I am restless.
The (flowery) stems of love are eternal. Waiting for this journey has made
  me tired.
Night and day my eyes search your face. Night and day my eyes look at
  your face.
Your face; my eyes.
Without you I am restless.

Safiya: First, I really love the quality of the music and the way it is sung by Nusrat Fateh Ali Khan. Second, I really became familiar with this song after my marriage. My husband was not with me for five months shortly after we married and that is why this song means so much to me.

MB: These words Safiya are very much about loving feelings. But now as I understand it some Quwalli songs are really devotional songs. Can you tell me something about what your Islamic faith means for you?

Safiya: I am a Muslim at heart but I don't pray five times a day and I don't listen to the Quwalli as a devotional song.

Wajiha explained that thinking of Quwalli songs as devotional songs is a perspective from an older generation. Traditional Quwalli singers have an almost harsh or punitive tone in their singing whilst Nusrat Fateh Ali Khan has almost fused the sound of Eastern and Western singing and younger people are drawn to this. Film music is also softening this traditional sound.

Both the traditional and modern Quwalli praise God but the modern Quwalli also has a human face. For younger educated people like Safiya and I, religion means that we make informed choices to balance our faith and our personal desire and liking to listen to music.

MB: Your son seems very delighted with music Safiya . . . what does he listen to?

Safiya: He listens to feeling songs . . . he likes the old-fashioned music, 1940s and 1950s. It was more lyric-based and he enjoys that.

MB: You write that Western music seems too loud and the words don't have much meaning for you . . . perhaps Indian music has more respect for the ears of the listener!?

MB: Some Indian music really has meaningful lyrics for me. But in Western music the lyrics seem very negative and not positive.

Wajiha remarked that some western lyrics at the moment are not at all encouraging. She noted that music influences us very strongly and wonders who is controlling all this negative hopeless sentiment.

MB: How do you think Indian lyrics differ from Western songs Safiya?

Safiya: I think Indian songs tell a story. Some say that you are not the saddest person in the world and the tell you how you can live your life in a more positive way . . . most are romantic songs . . . but most give hope . . . trust in God.

MB: Thank you Safiya, and Wajiha.

Roopa's writing

Music has always meant a lot to me. When I listen to music I usually experience different sensations depending on what I am listening to. In my school days around the age of 9 or 10 I was very fond of Western pop music. I had arrived here from India and this was the kind of music my friends listened to, so to merge into their circle I was interested in this kind of music too. However, as I grew through my teenage years I became genuinely fond of Western pop and rock music. It had excitement, energy and meant fun for me. Later I became more interested in the lyrics, looking out more for meaningful compositions not just a lot of noise.

In my search for more meaning in music I came across the British rock band, Queen, and I was deeply moved by many of their beautiful compositions. The flow of my own thoughts seemed to be captured and mirrored in certain songs like *The Show Must Go On* or *Who Wants to Live Forever?*. I listened to these compositions at an enquiring stage of my life when I had gone back to college in India and was very stressed while studying for my exams.

While I was deep in thought lots of spiritual questions arose for me. The essence of it all was that I was fussing about an exam when life itself was just a game. At the end of it all no worldly achievement would have everlasting impact or value. I heard similar things in certain songs by Queen and it was as if I had found a friend in those songs because I felt comforted. I then began to wonder how a successful rich Western rock band could have these thoughts about the purpose of life or the emptiness of life in general. This music is so moving for me.

It was at this time that I realised the importance of music for me. When I listened to it, it was as if I was living in a world of my own so much so that I was sometimes unaware of my surroundings. As time went on I outgrew this type of music but I still listened to it sometimes. I had also found the answers to some of my spiritual questions and become more mature, and didn't feel that I needed to seek a companion in music any more. I can be comforted by certain compositions by Queen but to relax I listen to South Indian classical music now.

During the past two years I have listened to a lot of South Indian classical music. Years ago I used to loathe it but now I am immensely fond of it. During my spiritual journey I came to understand the depth of Indian music in general. I am from the state of Kerala in South India and classical music there is very much associated with the temples. During festivals it is common for musicians to perform concerts in the temple grounds. So my journey into deeper spirituality meant a deeper and closer association with Indian classical music. Also, during the course of my spiritual journey, I was fortunate to visit the ashram of the great spiritual master in South India, Sri Sai Baba. As I became deeply influenced by his teachings, I understood more about devotion and I started listening to devotional music. Western music just did not fit well with this. Although most South Indian classical music is in the state languages which I don't understand I still love listening to it, there is something divine and spiritual about it.

I can still tune in easily to the mood of most kinds of music especially Indian film music which I have really enjoyed over the last 10 years. In particular I like the film songs in the Malayalam language, that is the official language of the state of Kerala in South India. These lyrics I understand. The film songs are influenced by Western rock music or they can have a North Indian classical flavour or an Islamic influence. The lyrics can be silly, happy, sad or a bit like poetry. This depends on the story in the film. I listen for the meaning of what the poet is talking about and if it has a personal meaning for me.

Music will always have a place of supreme importance in my life. I listen to South Indian classical music before I go to sleep. It calms the mind. The musical compositions are all dedicated to the Hindu deities. One composition might be about the Lord Ganesh while another may be about the Lord Krishna. If music was taken away from me it would mean a world of darkness, a mechanical dark world – unimaginable. Music for me is concerned with the meaning and beauty I seek.

Conversation with Roopa

MB: Roopa, you write that around the age of 10 when you came to England you were interested in Western pop music because of your school friends. Can you say more about that time?

Roopa: When I came to England I was not particularly interested in any kind of music. But my school friends influenced me and for their sake I became interested in Western pop music. But at age 13 I was not under their influence any more because I went back to India and I developed my own interest in Western music further. I listened to a lot of Western rock music then and became genuinely interested in it.

MB: I wonder, Roopa, if you are saying that your interest in 'pop' music at age 10 was more about how you could manage relationships with school friends?

Roopa: Yes it was. Now when I think back I realise that.

MB: So when you went back to India you brought with you Western 'rock' music. Were your friends in India interested in that?

Roopa: No they weren't so I kept it to myself . . . it was quite a lonely time.

MB: You remained in India until you were 29 . . . but at 18 or 19 you particularly enjoyed Queen songs. Is that right?

Roopa: Yes it is. I liked especially *The Show Must Go On* and *Who Wants to Live Forever?*.

MB: What was it in this music that so attracted you?

Roopa: What attracted me was the lyrics. There were questions in my mind which seemed to match these lyrics . . . questions about life . . . and they were a dramatic and colourful band. I first came across these songs when I first began to ask myself "Who wants to live forever?" and what would mankind's destiny be after he has lived his life in his physical body? . . . and I was surprised when I heard these songs that other people could ask these questions. I was also amazed that such a person as the lead singer of this band could think about something like that . . . something negative like that.

MB: Is this perhaps because he was the lead singer in this very rich Western band and didn't need to think like that?

Roopa: Yes . . . what made him think like that? This started questions in my mind and this went hand-in-hand with the spiritual enquiries which were going on for me at the same time.

MB: And from this self-questioning you arrived at the belief that no worldly achievement could have any real lasting value?

Roopa: Yes . . . before I listened to these songs I used to ask myself these questions about life and feel a bit negative about the answers. After I listened to them it helped me understand that other people had these questions too . . . so I had found a companion in these songs. Also it is an ultimate truth that nobody lives forever. No matter what you do or make in this life, unless it bears good deeds, you cannot take it with you after you pass away. This made me a bit sad and started many questions in my mind.

MB: It is interesting that you say that nothing lasts except good deeds . . . good deeds have this lasting value for you?

Roopa: Yes . . . Hinduism does not believe in this one life only . . . it teaches reincarnation and that a person's birth as an animal, or an insect, bird, or another human being or a higher being is entirely dependent on his or her actions which we call 'karma'. So good deeds bring forth good fruit . . . otherwise one's actions don't. That is why I say that you can only take the results of good deeds with you when you die.

MB: Thank you for that Roopa. You go on to write that you no longer feel the need to be comforted by listening to the music of Queen. Can you say something about the experience of listening to South Indian music?

Roopa: Before I became deeply interested in Karnatic music, that is South Indian classical music, I started listening to devotional music as a result of visiting my guru in South India, Sri Sai Baba. At the ashram I also heard instrumental music played in the South Indian classical style and it had a big impact on me there. South Indian classical musical compositions are dedicated to the Hindu gods. When I came back I attended religious music sessions and my interest grew further. So when I listen to South Indian classical music I automatically connect it to spiritual matters.

MB: But there is something special about this music isn't there?

Roopa: Yes . . . when I listened to the Queen music it made me happy. But now when I think back about it there was also something negative in it because it used to make me feel sad too sometimes . . . because if I want to see that singer again I can't because he's gone. His music is recorded but he is not there anymore. So what happened to him was just the fate of mankind. There is that emptiness in it. Although the music comforted me because somebody had thought the same things as me, it didn't give me ultimate happiness. But after my spiritual questions were answered I started listening to calming devotional music and I found that South Indian music has a fullness in it. Western music made me happy for a time but there was an emptiness in it.

MB: Yes . . . yes . . . that somehow there was an end of things?

Roopa: Yes . . . this was the end . . . a negativity about it.

MB: And you don't have that feeling when you listen to Indian classical music?

Roopa: No . . . it just satisfies my soul.

MB: Indian classical music has words Roopa, but you don't understand them. This doesn't seem to be an obstacle for you?

   Roopa went on to describe the strangeness of this in that although she doesn't follow all the words of the compositions she has an awareness that they are devotional. They are dedicated to the deities and this music is played in the temples. When she was in the ashram of Sri Sai Baba, compositions from North India and South India were played with very different languages so the words do not matter to her. It was the music.

MB: So it is the music itself . . . to my very Western ears it sounds as if there is much repetition.

Roopa: Yes, that's the way they sing it. I don't know much about it . . . I just love to listen to it . . . I haven't tried to study it.

MB: But this repetition does have an effect on the listener?

Roopa: Yes . . . a calming effect.

MB: Am I pushing this too far by saying that there is a kind of prayer feel about this repetition? (I was thinking particularly of the repetition in the saying of the *Rosary* – a devotional prayer in the Roman Catholic Church).

Roopa: Yes, I do feel that that the repetition is prayerful but along with this the texture of the music becomes more and more complex. It makes me realise how gifted these singers are to go into this complexity of notes and music and how this is a gift given by the divine.

MB: What is very interesting Roopa is that when you returned to India from England when you were 13, which must have been a difficult time for you, you brought back Western 'pop' music and you weren't concerned then about the lyrics of the songs in the Malayalam language, your home language, that were sung round about you. It didn't seem to reach you or connect with you then. But you do listen to Indian film music now in this language, the language you were born into.

Roopa: Absolutely . . . since my mid-20s I have listened to a lot of Malayalam film music and lyrics . . . this music expresses what it is to live in this part of the world.

MB: It sounds to me Roopa that your interest in music has described a kind of journey?

Roopa: Yes . . . yes that's right.

MB: And what is important for you now is whether you have found out something of importance on your musical journey?

Roopa: Yes I would absolutely agree because now I realise I am far more Indian than I thought I was. I tried to be Western at an early age because I thought that would be the right thing to do to be fashionable, but now I am much more Indian than I dreamed I ever would be. And if somebody had told me I would change so much I would never have believed them. I am more rooted in my country's language and everything now.

MB: And music seems to reflect that for you?

Roopa: And maybe I discovered a lot of who I really am through music.

Ubacharamulanu, composed by Thyagaraja and sung by Maharajapurum Santhanam

---

MB: In the piece of music you have chosen Roopa, *Ubacharamulanu*, there is vocal music and also complex rhythmic playing on the drum. Can you say something about this experience?

Roopa: This particular piece with the complex drum rhythms, I like it a lot. It reminds me of the temples and it has a particularly calming effect on me. I don't know the words but the singer is praising a deity in the music. He has used the *Raga Bhairavi* to improvise (raga is a scale) and the piece is dedicated to Lord Rama.

MB: The singing has a rather hypnotic effect on me. How would you describe its effect on you?

Roopa: I would describe it the same way. This is what I mean by calming. Maybe because it is devotional. It's devotion to God and this makes me calm.

MB: I'm very interested that you listen to this before you go to sleep.

Roopa: Yes . . . it's become a habit. My brother is not too fond of it so the best time for me to listen to it is before sleep. It's only my mother and myself who are fond of it . . . it's a bit like a sleeping pill!!

MB: But there may be something else interesting here. You play this music just before you go to a state where you are no longer conscious . . . I'm talking here about sleep. And one could almost begin to think from what you are saying that these sounds help you to go within to this state inside you?

Roopa: Yes . . . it does.

MB: Perhaps you . . .

Roopa: Though it makes me happy most of the time, sometimes I'm not in the mood for it . . . maybe my mind is not so quiet. But I have discovered that this playing helps a lot with sleep.

MB: You tell me that your mother listens to this music?

Roopa: Yes, she has always listened it.

MB: You won't remember because you would have been a baby, but you might have been told that your mother listened to this music before you were born or while you were still a small baby?

Roopa: Yes, I have been told that she did listen to this sort of music from my early childhood onwards.

MB: And these sounds would have been around certainly.

Roopa: She sings herself and is fond of this music.

MB: What would she have sung to you as a baby Roopa?

Roopa: I asked her this and she says that she would have sung simple lullabies to me in my native language.

MB: And she would have sung to you to help you to go to sleep?

Roopa: Yes, she did.

MB: So where are you now with music Roopa?

Roopa: South Indian classical music is an inevitable part of my life . . . I want to take it with me wherever I go . . . I want to know more and more about it. I know the music is divinely inspired. I am fascinated . . . and I want to know where the composers got their ideas from.

MB: Thank you Roopa.

CHAPTER 8

Interview with Joyce Ellis and choristers of the Kinder Children's Choirs

Charlotte Coupland aged 17, Lizi Norma aged 16 and Stephen Johnson aged 13, are choristers in the Kinder Children's Choirs of the High Peak and each has written on what music means for them.

The founder director of the Kinder Children's Choirs is Joyce Ellis and the accompanist is Andrew Burr.

Charlotte's writing

My thoughts and sensations usually reflect the mood of the piece of music I am listening to at the time. Instrumental only music captures my thoughts more because when I listen to it I am engulfed by the pattern of the sound rather than listening to the lyric in vocal music. I can relax more listening to music without lyrics. I am engaged by both the emotional plot and the changing states of the musical flow. I can then relate these to particular feelings I have and situations in my life.

I first became aware of the importance of music for me in coping with death. Words of particular songs helped me manage this experience. They clarified my feelings, and reassured me as well as bringing me comfort.

The experience of music has changed for me over the years. When I was younger the tone of music didn't mean much to me because I had nothing much to relate it to. At that time my conscious experience of a wide range of feelings was limited. Now, however, the tone or ambience of a piece of music can trigger memory or provoke new thoughts.

Music is really important for me and it would be very strange to be without it. It is always there for me rather like a comfort blanket.

Lizi's writing

When I listen to music I experience a mixture of feelings depending on what the music is. Some really loud modern music stresses me out so I just turn it off. That, however, isn't usual. Most music relaxes me or makes me want to dance. (I also have dance classes.) When a song comes on the radio that I like it cheers me up and makes me feel happy and glad. One of my favourite pieces of music is the Flower Duet, from *Lakme* by Delius. It is on my *Opera Babes* CD and I play it over and over again. I feel I could never become bored with it.

Music has always been part of my life. I have grown up with it and it has always been important to me. I can remember being fascinated by all the different musical instruments when I went to hear *Peter and the Wolf* by Prokofiev at a very young age. When I was five, I started to play the recorder and I remember feeling proud to be part of a group of musicians. More recently, I was inspired to play the oboe when the Kinder Choir had done a couple of concerts with orchestras. I loved the sound of the oboe so much on these occasions that I was determined that one day I would play the oboe like that.

The sense of achievement and excitement that I had when I was small and playing the recorder has expanded as my knowledge has grown and I continue to learn more about music. I appreciate it more and more. Music is my life. I play the oboe and the piano and have singing lessons. I am also in three choirs and a church group. I listen to music constantly and as soon as I get up in the morning I turn on the radio or a CD in my room. My brothers are constantly playing the piano or their guitars so I often join in or sing along. My older brother, who is studying music at university next year has often said that hearing would be the last sense he would choose to lose because he loves music so much. I couldn't stand it if music was taken away from me because it makes up a very important part of my life and I hate silence.

Stephen's writing

My feelings when I listen to music depend very much on the type of music I am listening to. If it is a happy joyful song in a major key I think of a story to go with it in my head. This usually fits perfectly and I feel in turn that my life is happy and I have nothing to worry about. It is as though God is telling me that He loves me. If it is funny bouncey music, I feel as though I want to bounce with it.

My emotions can change with the music and I feel as though I have been taken into the music itself which I enjoy. This, however, doesn't work if the sound is all 'screamy' and 'garagey'. I find that experience boring and rough.

When I didn't know much about music I thought it was just meant for things like theme tunes and I couldn't give music any adjectives at all. I was still in primary school then, singing in assemblies and productions on stage. I think I was about six years old. But when I started learning more about music, words appeared to describe it and it all became clearer and easier for me to think about and talk about.

Listening to music or singing, it feels like light and brightness leading the way forward to my path ahead in life. I used to feel lonely sometimes but when music was around the loneliness disappeared. Music is like a best friend. Music has changed for me as I have become older. When I was young I thought that I was the only one affected by music. Now I realise that music affects many people.

I know now that music is what I want to be involved with but where to start? I feel it's very important that I am involved with it every single day. If it was taken away from me I feel as if I would want to die. For me it is just not allowed to disappear. I would be stuck with nothing and I wouldn't want that. Music is my life.

Conversation with Joyce Ellis and the Kinder Choir choristers

MB: Joyce, how did this great choir start?

Joyce: I think it started because I had had so much encouragement and so much excitement from being in a choir as a child growing up that that experience never left me. I worked through the choir system as a chorister and eventually became the accompanist and then the conductor of the Maia Girls Choir in my home town of Stockport. In the meantime I went to music college in Manchester at 18 to study piano, cello and voice. When I went to Glyndebourne Festival Opera I had to leave the choir behind. I then sang professionally for about 20 years.

I had always felt that I wanted to start something here in the High Peak when my husband and I moved here in the late seventies. I realised there was very little for children in the way of quality singing in rural areas and this idea of a children's choir was something I kept coming back to. So I did something about it. How I did it is another story!

MB: Can you say something about this other story?

Joyce: Well . . . yes. Very few people knew me in the area because I had been doing a lot of travelling with my singing career. But there was one lady who came to me for piano lessons and I spoke to her about my idea for starting a choir. At the same time I was teaching the children of a friend who himself was a teacher and I told him of how I wanted to get back into education, so he arranged for me to go into schools on a voluntary basis to do some singing classes. When I then spoke further to Rosie, who was my pupil, she suggested I spoke to her husband Denis Harding, who is now chairman of the choir trust. I went to see him. Denis is a self-made businessman and he is also what I call a man with a social conscience. He and Rosie have a trust called the Barnabas Trust which encourages people to get things going in the community. He listened to what I wanted to do – start a children's choir – but said that the trust couldn't really support anything which didn't yet exist . . . so I said point taken, I'll go and make it exist! I contacted the local press and schools and said that I wanted to start a choir. At first there was some suspicion because I wasn't known in the area . . . but eventually we got the publicity and people wrote in saying that their child wanted to be in the choir. I divided the boys and girls and we had 20 boys and 40 girls. We then had a meeting at Hayfield Primary School to talk to the parents about what I wanted to do. We started in June 1991 and after the summer holiday I was terrified that no one would come back again, but they did after the summer break and that was how it started and it's been going from strength to strength ever since.

MB: So it's been going for 12 years now?

Joyce: Yes . . . 12 years.

MB: And you don't hold auditions?

Joyce: Not at all!

MB: So how is the choir formed? . . . and how do you get these beautiful voices?

Joyce: At the very first choir rehearsal ever, I gave them a note to sing . . . a middle G . . . and all the variety of notes I heard!! My poor heart sank . . . I knew I wanted to teach young people to sing but I had no idea of the size of the problem. The first few months of rehearsal therefore were taken up more or less with learning how to pitch notes. Then somebody said why didn't I divide them up into those who can sing and those who can't, but I said 'None of them can sing' (much laughter from the choristers who were listening). The first year was difficult but at the end of that year we had a concert in Buxton Opera House which I put on with my own guarantee of £500 . . . it was a great occasion with the Mayor and Lord Lieutenant present. The young ones sang in unison and I managed to get the older ones singing in three parts.

MB: And by that time they were all singing in tune?

Joyce: No . . . not really . . . but the odd voice doesn't matter . . . everybody else disguises it . . . and it was amazing how it all came together. We had Pauline Tinsley share the concert with us. She was one of our top international sopranos. She sang Rusalka's *Song of the Moon* and she also sang Ivor Novello's *I Can Give You the Starlight* with the choir accompanying in the background in three parts. This was quite moving considering they were not the choir they are now. We also had the Manchester Boy's Chorus who were great role models for us . . . and we all finished the concert with Mary Stuart's Prayer from Donizetti's opera *Maria Stuarda* as a combined item. It was such an exciting occasion . . . The phone was ringing into the early hours and my husband and I couldn't go to bed and just sat up talking all night in the warm July air on the doorstep because the excitement was still there, and we began to realise that this was the beginning of something quite special. Then the phone calls started again at 8 o'clock in the morning. The year before this Denis had given me a grant of £1000 to get the choir started and I never needed to touch that £1000.

MB: Great.

Joyce: I originally wanted there to be no subscription for the choir members but I couldn't manage to sustain this.

MB: But how do you choose the choir?

Joyce: Well we don't choose. When new children come in they join the training group, then the junior or the boy's choir, by age and standard and then there is the concert choir which depends not only on age but on ambition, commitment and how you approach your singing. We therefore have the training choir, the junior and the boy's choir and then the concert choir which is the apex of the organisation. We also have a youth choir with the purpose of encouraging the boys who are in the changing voice stage. It is made up of the young baritones with some of the senior girls.

MB: What is the future for the choir?

Joyce: To keep creating opportunities for young people through singing, concerts, recordings, TV and radio, and tours and to continue to give them excitement, drama.

MB: There isn't very much in this area like this.

Joyce went on to reflect on this but also that what was so very special about a choir is that it didn't require a great individual talent to reach the top. If one was going to reach the top as a sportsman or a musician there had to be an enormous amount of individual talent but a mediocre talent could enjoy the benefits that the whole choir creates together, like the various travel experiences the choir has had and the CDs they have made together. Joyce would like this to continue but in order to do this it was of the utmost importance that their good standard should be maintained. As she said "If they don't maintain the standard they will not have the opportunities". This then brought the conversation round to how this standard was maintained. I decided to bring in the choristers at this point.

MB: How does Miss Ellis manage to get this great choir to sound the way it does?

Charlotte: Lots and lots of practice ... going over things but in a very structured way. For example we divide up the parts so that the harmonies do it first, then the sopranos and then we run through it together until we've caught up with everybody ... then we do another section in the same way ... then perhaps add it to the first section, do it without the copy ... then do a bit more ... then without the copy. We build it up like that so the learning isn't all at once. We then move on to doing it from memory.

MB: So you do it like that most of the time which means that there is a repeated structure to learning a new piece?

Charlotte: Yes ... it's good ... because everyone is different in how they learn things and I think this way is best because you are doing little bits at a time so your brain can take it in.

MB: And of course when you put the copy down you look where?

Charlotte (smiling): At Miss Ellis ... or we should be! When we had a rehearsal with the little ones the other day ... they hadn't sung with us before and they were looking all around them and behind them and Miss Ellis was trying her best to keep their attention, but it was a losing battle.

Joyce: I had to apologise to them that I wasn't Kylie Minogue or David Beckham or someone glorious and that they have had to put up with littl'ol'me and they're stuck with that!

MB: So what else about this sound you make?

Stephen: Well ... we have warm up ... we sing scales and exercises so that our voices are in tune and are placed. For instance, we use vowel sounds in the arpeggios and scales. We also practise consonants to develop the lip and tongue muscles.

Lizi: We also do breathing exercises. We work at how we stand how to project our voices. We have training weekends as well.

Charlotte: We have to be reminded a lot about the different things to do because we can concentrate so hard on one thing and forget to breathe at the right time for instance. You have to train yourself to think what you are doing all the time.

Stephen: When you do it a lot you do get used to it though, like breathing from the diaphragm, which really helps control your breath.

Lizi: It's really strange how this happens. We do exercises on feeling where the diaphragm is and how it moves. It's quite amazing. We did an exercise on holding each other's ribs and it's quite weird ... they move!!

Joyce told of an exercise where she tries to push the front row back into their seats by firmly pushing their diaphragms. If they are breathing and standing properly they might wobble on their feet but they don't sit back on their chairs!! We then talked about the words of the songs and how they are so clear. This was put down to a lot of work on consonants, the Ds and Ts. Charlotte commented that this was difficult work because a lot of young people are careless with their speech and the exercises sound funny but if they didn't do these exercises people can't hear what you're singing!! (One would hope that opera choruses and soloists would attend to this point more!!)

Joyce pointed out a bigger problem with words – almost a national difficulty. This is the disappearance of the 'th' sound. She feels it is going to disappear altogether and that some children have great difficulty with this particular pronunciation. She puts it down to a lazy tongue and said how they really have to work at this in rehearsals.

I asked how often they rehearsed.

Lizi: We rehearse twice a week unless there is a concert coming up at Christmas or in July. Then we have extra rehearsals.

Charlotte: But these extra rehearsals really pay off. When I was doing GCSEs last year, extra ones were put in for people who had missed a few and who needed to catch up with their part in the harmony.

MB: So it's a real commitment . . . you've got to get yourself organised and get to rehearsal . . . great. Are there butterflies before a concert?

Charlotte: Apprehensive really . . . you want to do your best for Miss Ellis and also people are paying to watch and listen . . . but you are also excited at the same time.

MB: At the concerts I have been to I was very impressed that everyone stood so completely still . . . tell me about this?

Lizi: Well we've been trained . . . very well!! (much laughter). Miss Ellis gets rid of fidgeting in the training choir. I remember when we were singing at the Buxton Opera House she was very firm and said something like, "If you can't sit with your legs still you can't sit on stage".

Joyce: Yes, I won't let anybody sit on the stage unless they can sit still . . . children aren't trained to sit still anymore . . . but at a performance they can't distract the audience and they can't distract the people who are performing. So right from the beginning of their training they must sit still . . . and this is hard for them.

I then asked each of them how old they were when they had joined the choir. Charlotte said she was a bit older than the others in that she started when she was 12. Her mum had always wanted her to be in the choir but she hadn't wanted to when she was younger. She knew some people who were in it when she was 12 and they were really interested so she joined. She added that it was her decision as well as her mum's. Lizi's friend Rachel had joined originally and came back saying how much she had enjoyed it. So, Lizi thought that she might like to have a go. She was seven or eight at the time and has been in the choir ever since. Then I asked Stephen when he had joined.

Stephen: Well . . . in my primary school I was in the choir because I was interested in singing and my teacher thought I was very good at it. So my mum thought I might give it a try. Eventually I made friends and thought this was a great team.

MB: So how old were you then?

Stephen: I was eight then and I've been singing with them ever since.

MB: Can you say something about your favourite piece of choir music and why it is important for you?

Stephen: The piece that really stands out for me is *Gospel Train* (Gwyn Arch's arrangement of a traditional song). I like it because we made sound effects along with the music and it's really like a train going forward . . . great fun!

Lizi: *Cantate Domino* (Rupert Lang) is my favourite piece. It's really fun to sing because at one point we all babble . . . we sing our own bit and improvise. And it's got fabulous harmonies. We've recorded it on the CD *Can You Hear Me?* and it sounds really good. When you're singing it you don't really hear all of it but if you're listening it sounds really great . . . wow!

Charlotte: I don't have one favourite piece. I think I like the themed concerts like *Broadway/Cowboy* (arranged by Andrew Burr) or *Les Miserables*. There are a lot of different pieces of music and solos as well and sometimes we do actions to them. This brings in the drama side of things and I like that.

Joyce added that they sometimes have two or three rehearsals with Stefan Janski who is Head of Opera Studies at the Royal Northern College of Music. He comes and personalises the music, brings in a little bit of movement, a little bit of step. This year they are doing some Gershwin songs and spirituals. However, the choristers also enjoy contributing their own moves to songs so that they can do it on their own!

MB: What has been your best or worst or most embarrassing experience in the choir? . . . be brave!

Charlotte: I really like singing in the Opera Galas where we have singers like Frances McCafferty . . . and we do it for one night only . . . you have someone different to learn from and there are different people in the audience. I like these concerts the best.

Lizi: It's hard to choose just one great experience because we have so many good opportunities. Last year we sang at the Commonwealth Games in Manchester and that was great. There are also the tours in Germany and we go as a family and all look after each other.

Stephen: I really like singing at the Buxton Opera House.

MB: Buxton is going to love you for that!

Stephen: But we also went to St Paul's in London for the millennium year and sang at the Children's Society Millennium Service and people came from all over the country . . . but I also remember a really embarrassing experience when I first joined the choir at about seven. It was my second rehearsal and I didn't know the words so Miss Ellis asked one of the choristers to get them for me. She said "Please would you get a *copy* for Stephen" and I said "I don't like coffee but I'll have tea".

MB: (A combined 'ah . . . poor thing' rose from the group).

Joyce: I have an embarrassing story. It was our very first concert at the Buxton Opera House. I was very nervous about the concert, trying to focus on all aspects of the evening, looking after the little ones, answering all the questions from choristers at my dressing room door, trying to remember how I would introduce guests and talk about items in the programme plus a hundred and one other things . . . there were so many things going on in my head. I got changed into my finery to go on stage, but when I came off at the interval I realised I was wearing my slippers instead of my posh high heels . . . so what a picture!

MB: Lizi . . . you want to say something?

Lizi: I think really that it's important to say that even though we have to work very very hard and sometimes we get tired and very nervous before a concert, when we go on stage and sing it's such a wonderful experience to see people really enjoying the music that we make . . . it's really great. At the end of the concert at Buxton we sometimes get a standing ovation and I really feel so proud to be part of the choir. You get such a wonderful thrill at the concert that it makes the hard work leading up to it really worthwhile . . . it's an amazing experience to be in the choir.

MB: Thank you very much indeed. Joyce what is your best experience conducting the choir?

Joyce: There are so many good experiences, but the one that is always with me is standing up in front of the choir and seeing it as a musical instrument. They are a fabulous group of people who go off and are individuals who live their own lives but when they come together on stage all these persons suddenly become one instrument and sometimes standing up there can be quite nerve wracking. Have the rehearsals gone well . . . or how do I feel personally that day? . . . but sometimes there are moments of great electricity and perhaps it's at these times we are creating better music than we have done before. Somehow everyone is more alive, more inspired and all of this comes together to create something special, where the mood or the emotion is more intense. It doesn't happen all the time because that's when it's genius and genius doesn't happen all the time.

MB: A special moment?

Joyce: But there has to be a standard which the performance and the singing don't drop below . . . but when these moments of genius occur it's very special and very moving and we've had a few of these. Also we've had young people who have come into the choir who have not been able to pitch or would not have had any singing voice at all if they hadn't come and had the choir experience. They would never have learned to pitch and sing in tune or find a singing sound in their voices . . . they would have missed all that opportunity. And to see them standing up and enjoying the concert, enjoying the experience and being fulfilled . . . without the Kinder Choir that would never have happened perhaps . . . that is very special and just as important as the great performance. This of course would not have happened for children if they had tried to join a choir in which they had had their voices tested beforehand. And I must say that most of the children in the Kinder Choir would not be here if that had been the requirement. That's special for them and for me . . . to come and make music with everybody so that we can create that special electricity together. I always tell them they can't do it without me but of course I can't do it without them . . . it's a partnership.

MB: Thank you Joyce . . . Where are you three going with music from now on?

Lizi: Music is a big part of my life now . . . I play the piano and the oboe so I'll definitely carry on with it. I shall probably go to university so I'd like to find a choir and I'll keep playing the piano and the oboe. Most of the time outside school I'm involved with music.

Charlotte: I'd like to carry on with music because it's introduced me to all sorts of different experiences in my life. Starting later with music it just feels like a beginning and I want to do more and more of it.

MB: Stephen?

Stephen: Well I reckon music *is* my life. The choir has shown me that music is something I really want to be part of . . . so I also want to go on with singing in opera.

MB: Tell me a bit more about this Stephen.

Stephen: Well I've been doing some work with Opera North and it's great fun even though I'm at school. I've played Harry a cheeky boy in Britten's *Albert Herring* and Jano in Janacek's *Jenufa* also the First Boy in the *Magic Flute* by Mozart . . . I'm a bit more confident on stage now.

MB: Do you have a picture of where you might want to go in your career?

Stephen: Yes I do . . . I would like to be a big opera star.

MB: That's wonderful.

Joyce: We just hope that a decent instrument reappears after Stephen's voice changes . . . because he's just on the verge of it now. He's had a wonderful treble career so far . . . he's won festivals and sung solos. But what is so special about a boy's voice is that it's fleeting but we do hope that his voice reappears in just such a great form, Stephen is philosophical about it.

Stephen: It's just part of life . . . we can't do much about it.

MB: We are all keeping our fingers crossed for you Stephen. Thank you all very much.

The Kinder Children's Choirs of the High Peak

Founder director   Joyce Ellis
Accompanist   Andrew Burr

     Kinder Collection
     Cantique de Kinder
     Can you hear me?
     Christmas with Kinder

These are all available in CD (£12) or cassette (£8) plus postage.

e-mail: www.kinder.childrenschoirs@ukgateway.net

CHAPTER 9

Interview with
The Reverend David Hart

David is an Anglican priest and Senior lecturer in Theology and Religious Studies at King Alfred's College, Wincester. He is Secretary to the World Congress of Faiths and on the steering committee of the Sea of Faith. He divides his time between Britain and India.

David's writing

Music is a collection of linguistic signs which appeal to the sense of hearing , and help us make sense of our lives through the exploration of our emotions, and to a lesser extent our intellect. I would find the full appreciation of the world of meaning to be very difficult indeed without the world of music.

A lot in life is difficult to express in words because there is so much ambivalence: running through Yeats' writing is the sea as a symbol of the ever-shifting ambivalence of life and a lot of that ambiguity is for me better expressed in music; Mozart, for example, knows the joys of seduction (*Don Giovanni*) and also the heights of religious ecstasy (*Ave Verum*), while Mahler and Bruckner have passages of sea-like pervasive movement of emotion. The music for me is furthered by 'programme notes' which explain much of the impetus and background for the writing of the music: Mahler and Britten, for instance, wrestled very much with the question of their social and sexual identities and their music was an expression of the struggle.

I think the verbal stories are what make opera perhaps for me the highest form of music ... appealing to both the verbal and the tonal, word and music, composers like Verdi and Puccini are unsurpassable in depth of joy. I recently heard Puccini's *Messa di Gloria* and am fascinated with the idea of an 'operatic divine service' incorporating our emotions but also involving the whole gathered religious community in an act of participation; this brings even more of our senses, intellectual, credal and emotional, into the picture.

Mahler's *Fifth Symphony* is poignant because I heard it alongside the film *Death in Venice* and alongside the agony and the ecstasy of my own 'gay' sensitivity, and realise something of the exclusion the artist feels from family and society, something that cannot in the nineteenth century be adequately conveyed in words at all, and which the poignancy of the agonised music helps the listener to perceive something of the isolation and the vision of physical beauty that comes through such an existential isolation from its source and inspiration.

I remember when my mother died of cancer in her 50s Wagner's *Tristan and Isolde*, the death scene, enabled me to make some connection to my own situation that enabled the tears to flow where nothing or no one else alleviated my pain.

Conversation with David

MB: David ... your writing is an account of a very adult experience of music. Could you say something about when you first became interested in music?

David: Yes, well it's difficult to remember the first conscious piece of music but I think it probably was that tune on the radio, which is all we had in the early 50s, which was the *Listen with Mother* tune.

MB: And were there any particular pieces of music after that?

David: Well, what happened then was that I joined the choir aged about six or seven, the Anglican church choir, and I got interested in music and it turned in a more classical direction, I suppose ... I always used to enjoy the anthems in particular. There were the service settings which were the bread and butter, but the anthems and the sort of exotic names of people like Herbert Howells and others stuck in my mind. And as a soprano one wanted to try to get to the top notes and I admired the other boys who were able to do it in a better way than me ... I only became deputy head chorister, not head chorister. I don't think I did have a very beautiful voice but I did enjoy that experience and that was about between 6 and 14 ... I think there was a lot of formation of my musical appreciation at that time.

MB: That was English church music?

David: Yes, in the main stream Anglican tradition.

MB: So that's between 6 and 14 ... and after then?

David: Well from 15 to 18 I was swatting to get to Oxford to do originally English literature, then I changed to theology. But I think that the music that then became quite important for me was Tchaikovsky ... the symphonies and the *First Piano Concerto* which I played on record ... I didn't have much time to go to the choir then so it was really much more private listening at home in Bromley, Kent.

MB: And then you went to Oxford?

David: And in a way that was the opening up of things because there was the glorious caviar of concerts in the evening ... and I went to Keble College ... which had a wonderful chapel ... there was a lot of religious music there and also that was the first time I went to opera at the Playhouse and the New Theatre and so much was a delight. I took to it like a duck to water, though not as a practitioner but as an appreciator.

MB: It would be a wonderful place to experience all of this?

David: Absolutely ... yes. The Holywell music room and everything.

MB: David ... you bring in the faith aspect of your experience of music when you write of the idea of an operatic divine service inclusive of our emotions and the religious community in an act of participation. Would this reflect your position as an active member of the Sea of Faith and how is it that you find a place there?

David: Yes ... I mean to be honest I think that quite a lot of my operatic sense probably comes more from a root in the Anglican Church, where at Oxford at Keble College I was very much under the influence of the Anglo Catholic Movement in which the beauty of worship, the vestments, the incense, the music, the architecture ... themselves as well as the Word sort of widened one's understanding and one's perception of spiritual things ... The Sea of Faith is a rather wordy organisation. But it is rather a paradoxical situation because these are people who have become unhappy with the traditional words of churches and are trying to reformulate their understanding and perception of what has been known as the transcendent ... but the groups who try to do this tend to use words. Some of us feel that that is not exhaustive of the task and that what we are talking about here is a possible other way of coming to engage with the problem of the transcendent.

MB: There is a problem with words isn't there?

David: Yes, it's a problem with interpretation. But if we learn the subtleties of intonation and the different word families and groupings and if we can perceive that and share that in the best possible sense as human beings, if we can learn that together, then those subtleties do make language the best way of communicating. But it is an art and a skill which we don't just land in by our birth and there is a dumbing down of language which is rather difficult ... probably in the musical world too and therefore I think the sensitivities and the philosophy do need to be often articulated and discussed as we are doing now.

MB: Returning to your writing ... do you consider music as a link to the word – the verbal ... is music perhaps the prime source of emotional engagement?

David: Yes, it's a question I have wrestled with quite a lot in my personal and spiritual life and in my academic and theological work, what is the primal linguistic structure? I think that as a disciple of Don Cupitt and an interpreter of religion from a non-realist perspective ...

MB: That would be a Sea of Faith position?

The Sea of Faith holds the view that there is no God out there. God is a product of our own minds. He, She or It is a mental construct, the non-realist position.

In order not to confuse this mental construct of God totally with who I am as a human being, the usual process is to project God out there. It is the most convenient way of talking or thinking about He, She or It.

David: That would be a Sea of Faith position. I would have to say that the broad-brush stroke of that philosophical position would follow Wittgenstein's understanding that language, human language, the linguistic structure is the ultimate nature of our meaning as human beings and we can't get beyond that. And that does seem to have a focus on words as being the most important but of course music is another linguistic structure equally subtle, so there is a question as to whether there is a primal musical structure or something else like body language and I am not sure what the answer to that is . . . although I've got an intuition that as humans beings the linguistic structure is the profoundest way we communicate together.

MB: Mmn . . . you wouldn't consider music as a pre-linguistic phenomenon?

David: Yes . . . I think in some senses it might be although with 'pre' and 'post' there is a little value judgement put in. If 'pre' meant it wasn't as sophisticated a form then clearly I don't want to say that but you could say that it is trying to come to words; obviously that happens in opera and it happens in Mahler for example, as you know there are parts of his symphonies that have words in, so it sort of comes into words . . . I think it is a spectrum more than anything else.

MB: Yes . . . and perhaps the first example of this spectrum happens when we are babies. The baby's cry, as Anthony Wilden[1] writes, says everything, whilst when we come to words proper we begin to say one thing or another. So . . .

David: Yes, and I think intonation, which we have mentioned before and which perhaps the Sea of Faith and Don Cupitt haven't looked at very much, but the intonation of how you say things . . . for example you can say **Fire** or *fire* and that can make a lot of difference and that is the kind of subtlety that music is based on.

MB: And Susanne Langer[2] writes that a particular sweep and intensity of phrase in music would equally fit the words 'O joy' or 'O horror'.

David: Absolutely.

MB: The same musical phrase carrying different meanings . . . yes.

David: And I think that in so far as the Sea of Faith would want to discover ambivalence, in religious poetry and dogma, the notion that you can't speak directly of God; such an interest in intonation should be of importance here.

David and I went on to discuss programme notes at concerts and he maintained that such written information added to his enjoyment of what he was about to listen to and reading such information honoured the composer in that one should be properly prepared to listen to the music knowing the context from which it came.

We then turned to the Adagietto from Mahler's *Fifth Symphony* and I talked about it being used in the film *Death in Venice*, an adaptation of the story by Thomas Mann. I reminded him that he had read *Death in Venice* around the time of listening to Mahler's music.

MB: Remembering when you heard this music, you write of the sharp heightened sense of isolation and awareness of the vision of physical beauty and this physical beauty being unattainable. Could you say something more about this?

David: Yes ... as you were asking the question then there was certainly a very vivid recollection of my own emotion when I was about 23. But I suppose the intellectual person that comes to mind is Plato ... because it does seem to me that the whole idea of desire for the beautiful and the other virtues is inevitably linked with our physical desire and Plato was someone who understood that, without making the value judgements that Christianity later made on the top of Plato. For myself it's very important to understand music such as the Mahler movement as being about embodied persons and the programme notes of Mahler are made very specific by Visconti in the film *Death in Venice*. They are very much focused on sexual desire which is of course fairly frequent in the musical, artistic and intellectual world and, yes, I feel an identity with that and, yes, I feel an identity with the isolation that particular forms of sexuality put the individual in and also the longing for completion and understanding in the spiritual sense ... so sexuality and spirituality are inherently connected I think when we come to this phase of my musical appreciation and of my life.

David then went on to talk of his interest in India with which he became aquainted in his 30s when he was a chaplain at Loughborough University in 1990 and where he met the local Indian community. He talked of his experience of India as having a symbolic maternal role for him after the death of his mother. The music of India was important to him because he was entranced by it as he heard it in the several temple festivals and noted that in trying to find recordings of the music was told politely that they didn't do that sort of thing, i.e. recordings. He finds the music haunting but does not feel that he is really attuned to it yet and would like to learn more, but this is where he is at the moment musically.

MB: You say that you don't feel quite at home yet in the music of India?

David: In a way that's an interesting question because I wouldn't like to feel at home with any music and this is what we have been talking about.

MB: Feeling not at home?

David: And feeling that one's life ... is a journey and I don't know what the next chapter is ... how long the Indian chapter will last. I know I'm not going to go back to the intensity of Tchaikovsky when I was 18 ... that in a curious way was a high point even more than the Mahler symphony but I know that intensity will never come again ... I know that ... but there may be more of Wordsworth's 'reflection in tranquility', that sort of thing, who knows. There are composers who are closed books to me whom I would like to learn more about and enjoy.

The Adagietto – the fourth movement from Mahler's *Fifth Symphony*

MB: Perhaps we can look at the Adagietto now. It can stand on its own, as they say, or it can be heard as part of the whole symphony.

David: It stands on its own in the film but if I've got time I prefer to listen to the whole symphony so that one builds up to it as it were. I think it does stand on its own in terms of what I've been talking about. It's a very haunting piece of music isn't it really?

MB: and very yearning?

David: Absolutely . . . and it's difficult to see the form of it and that is partly why I came to love Mahler in my middle 20s because the form is difficult to specify . . . but yet it's in movement . . . and it's rather like . . . the symbol of the sea which was very important for Yeats because he saw the tide coming in and out as a very vivid symbol of the increasing ambivalence of life and of the waves of positive and negative emotion of joy and sorrow . . . Mahler speaks of this for me better than any other composer.

MB: I often think of Mahler as the composer of the unconscious, as if he presents the flow of his unconscious before us without tidying it up.

David: That's interesting . . . I haven't thought of that but I see what you mean and also you can't specify whole areas of his music . . . Yes.

We then went on to discuss the shape of the Adagietto in that it wasn't nice and tidy and didn't have clear differentiation between one part and another. It could be described broadly as ABA in form but again the boundaries are unclear. It was felt to be more an organic movement. David also commented that the themes link up movements, the same theme appearing in different movements, and that is why listening to the whole symphony gives most satisfaction.

The first two movements of Mahler's *Fifth Symphony* are an obsession with death. The first movement is a funeral march and the second has strong angry bitter passages. The Scherzo, the third movement, stands alone – very ebullient. The fourth movement, the Adagietto, is for strings and harp only and is calm, serene, at times yearning and then resigned. It is very beautiful, leading to the optimistic fifth movement, the Rondo. David remarked . . .

David: It is very beautiful but it is about fate. The symphony starts, as in the *Death in Venice* story, with the fact of death. Venice is being swallowed up by the plague of cholera. Also, in the Thomas Mann story, within an individual life there are lots of links being made between the discovery of sexuality and mortality, that to some extent they go together. The sexual project is almost inevitably doomed. This is shown for me in this Mahler movement and pushes me to discovering this in my personal relationships more vividly now than in previous stages in my life. It may be more poignant for the gay person in our society to actually realise the unattainability of that vision of beauty and perfection in a single life.

MB: Could you say a bit more of what this beauty is about?

David: Yes ... it was Nietzsche who said something to the effect that Eros was given poison to drink by the Christians. He didn't die of it but he degenerated into vice. I think what Eros means in Greek thought is ... as well as being able to create children one can create an opera, a work of art, and the basic human energies are almost infinitely malleable which is a frightening thought isn't it? The great artists are often very incomplete people because they have put their whole life into one pursuit of the beautiful and they are inevitably not going to reach it so they are unhappy whether they are Mahler or Van Gogh. It is difficult to judge them because they teach us so much about the spiritual quest ... this movement is also about yearning ... what are they yearning for? I think Jung gets the closest to this when he uses the term integration of the male and female, the animus and anima ... not only in the outside life but also in the inner self. Every person has an inner male and female aspect and you have to find the balance of them within your own psyche as well as in the outside world ... and to actively reach that integration, that sense of spirituality, is a lifetime task according to Jung ... I've seen and admired it from time to time in people over 80 in India and also in the West but it's very very rare that one reaches this state. One of the Platonic people who understands this is Iris Murdoch who focuses quite a lot in her books on the pure young artists and young people who try to reach that perfect vision of integration but who destroy themselves or others on the way either by broken emotional relationships or literally by death.

MB: You talk about a quest, the yearning towards integration of the male and female, a kind of spirituality, but one that seems to be difficult to define further than this?

David: Yes ... definition is fencing us in ... we don't need to be fenced in. Too often traditions fence us in and tell us we can't stray beyond, and that's unnecessary ... it stunts our movement and spiritual growth as creatures of God or whoever created us ... or if nothing created us. As human beings we wish to explore and as long as we don't do harm to others we should explore different forms of language and understanding and communication ... that's the meaning of life.

MB: Thank you David.

References

Wilden A (1972) *System and Structure*. Tavistock Publications, London, p. 24.
Langer S (1953) *Feeling and Form*. Routledge and Kegan Paul, London.

Further reading

Arnold M (1933) Dover Beach. In: *The Albatross Book of Living Verse*. Collins and Company, London. The poem Dover Beach refers to the 'sea of faith' and its ebb and flow.

Boulton D (1996) *A Reasonable Faith: introducing the Sea of Faith Network*. Sea of Faith Network, 15c Burton Street, Loughborough LE11 2DT.

Magee B (1987) *The Great Philosophers*. BBC Books, London. A history of philosophy from Plato to the present day. Nietzsche and Wittgenstein are among those discussed.

CHAPTER 10

Interview with Dr Margaret

Dr Margaret is a busy general practitioner in a medical practice in Derbyshire.

Dr Margaret's writing

I listen to music in different ways at different times. Sometimes I need to manipulate my mood. For example, I may want to lift my mood or relish the opportunity to wallow in melancholy. At times I will opt to choose to listen to specific pieces in my collection, for example the Mendelssohn *Violin Concerto*, the Saint-Saens *Organ Concerto* or the *Messiah*, then at other times it could be perhaps the Elgar *Cello Concerto* some Schubert lieder or the Mozart *Requiem*. More frequently now I go with the flow and just listen to whatever is on Classic FM, for instance, which relaxes my mood when I'm travelling home from work.

I like to get completely lost in the music too on some occasions that is, when given the opportunity to fully relax, but this does not happen often because my own thoughts intrude a lot. English twentieth century music is my escape music. Delius' *First Cuckoo in Spring*, Vaughan Williams' *Fantasia on a Theme by Thomas Tallis* or the *Five Variants of 'Dives and Lazarus'* are favourites.

My earliest memories of enjoying music are travelling in the car on long journeys and singing 'I'll sing you one–o', and making up, our own words to Schubert's *The Trout*. Singing in the school choir and the church choir and enjoying carol singing from the age of six are also fond early memories. Then, a little later, rummaging in my great aunt's piano stool and a feeling of amazement that the written note could be translated into sound, this comes to mind around that time as well. An experience which stands out at that time was starting piano lessons aged seven with 'Madame', I think her surname may have been Smith, who had blue glasses and yellow hair! The names of the lines of the bass stave GBDFA and the treble stave spaces FACE are indelibly imprinted in my mind, so I learned something! Also there was the thrill of moving my hands about the keyboard and good sounds coming out sometimes. One interesting later moment I remember was my father telling me to put more feeling into my piano playing. I would have been about 10 or 11, so maybe I was just a little too young for that. My father was very moved by music but had never had the opportunity to play.

Classical music has become more important in my life over the last eight years in that it has proved therapeutic at a time of emotional upheaval after my marriage ended. Initially I manipulated what I listened to in order to provide a safety net, a holding container, for my emotions. With the passage of time, however, I'm now able to enjoy the roller-coaster of feelings caused by certain music.

Participating in music and gaining proficiency when young gave me a sense of achievement. As I grew older my playing did become more expressive and I became more moved when listening to music. Unfortunately the only instrument I have played has been the piano and I wish I had had the opportunity to play another instrument and perhaps the chance to make music in a small ensemble or orchestra. However, I did enjoy playing piano duets.

I have two children and my experience of music has broadened over the years. As they have grown and learned to play instruments, one piano and flute and the other piano, oboe and saxophone, I have naturally become interested in their playing and more aware of woodwind playing in general. Music that they have played in the past has become of great significance to me. Pieces include Handel's *Music for the Royal Fireworks* and Britten's Pan from *Six Metamorphoses after Ovid*. These pieces have become better than photographs for me as I can now picture and hear them playing at the same time.

I also now sing in a group which performs a varied programme two or three times a year. My girls are generally in the orchestra which accompanies us which makes the experience extra special. Through participating in this music society I have become familiar with works previously unknown to me, for example Brahms' *German Requiem*.

I have also become interested in jazz. I enjoy listening to it although I don't know much about it. However, I particularly admire the ability and courage of those who improvise. I have always enjoyed the ballet but I also have become more interested in opera recently. I think I love the spectacle and the emotional intensity.

Music is very important in my life. It can uplift me or let me be reflective. I listen to music first thing in the morning, when I'm driving, and last thing at night. I often fall asleep still listening! Hearing loss would be very hard for me to bare. I think, maybe, I could cope with visual loss more easily.

Conversation with Margaret

MB: Margaret . . . you write that you listen to music in different ways. Can you say something about the pieces which lift your mood and those which allow you to wallow, as you say?

Margaret: I think that Baroque music uplifts me and I particularly enjoy *Zadok the Priest* by Handel. It must have been a most wonderful experience to be sitting in the audience for the first performance, listening to the gentle opening in the strings and suddenly this tremendous sound of the voices bursting upon you . . .

I'm sure the audience was not expecting that . . . it still makes the hair on the back of my neck stand on end when I hear it. There are also a lot of pieces in the *Messiah* that have the same effect on me. I think there is a joy about these pieces.

MB: There is a brightness about them isn't there?

Margaret: Yes, they feel very clear, like a sunny Spring day. More recent music can also be very uplifting like Elgar's *Pomp and Circumstance March*.

MB: Yes in the concert hall the big build-up to the main melody . . . it really is an experience of the blood surging through the veins.

Margaret: Yes . . . and at a calmer level, Mozart's *Marriage of Figaro* and the *Magic Flute* . . . they are so bright and cheerful and have a clarity of writing . . . I think perfect is the word to describe them.

MB: I am interested in your use of the word clarity. You've used it twice now in your description of music and it does seem to hold importance for you. I'm quite heartened that you as a GP put such store on clarity.

Margaret: Well in a sea of mud and murky waters it is good to experience something fresh and clear. I think there are times for murky music but I enjoy the clarity.

MB: Yes.

Margaret: In opera, there is Rossini's *William Tell* and the *Barber of Seville*. These are both sparkly and similar to Mozart in clarity. More modern compositions, such as Prokofiev's *Peter and the Wolf* or *Romeo and Juliet*, I enjoy for the same sorts of reason.

MB: Yes, I hadn't thought about that thread of clarity running through. I think that is a very interesting expression to use of music through its different periods. Which pieces then Margaret allow you to wallow?

Margaret: My big favourite would be the Elgar *Cello Concerto*.

MB: Yes, yes.

Margaret: I always feel a bit self-indulgent in letting myself wallow in it . . . but it is so beautiful and moving . . . at the end I sort of feel like a bit of wet lettuce. But sometimes . . .

MB: Sometimes it's OK to feel like a bit of wet lettuce . . . yes? This suggests to me that you give music a very important place in your life. You can choose to engage with it . . . and use it and you are in control of the choosing?

Margaret: Yes . . . I don't feel as if I have to listen to music all the time . . . I simply can't.

MB: Of course not. It would seem to be the only available place for you to take 'time out' as it were, given the demands of being a busy GP. You can't ever get lost there!

Margaret: Yes ... my time commitment to the practice is increasing and also my commitments to the family. I enjoy reading but I find that I fall asleep after a few pages so I don't tend to get anywhere with my book and it doesn't seem to give me what I need. I can just opt in and out of music without having to remember what has gone before. I can switch off and I don't have to concentrate. I just let it flow over me most of the time.

MB: Yes ... this is interesting about music ... that to enjoy it ... you can just experience it. Some people concentrate on music very hard but it is also a medium in which you don't need to concentrate at all and you can still enjoy it enormously?

Margaret: Yes, absolutely ... I really do feel this.

MB: Yes, there are all sorts of ways of listening.

Margaret then went on to describe how she listens in a more concentrated way at weekends. She recently attended a Schubert concert recital of *Die Schöne Mullerin* (*The Maid of the Mill*) where there was a pre-concert talk and she says that she felt able to appreciate much more of the performance because of it. I reminded her that Schubert wasn't a new composer for her in that she used to sing *The Trout* in the car when she was a child. She added that Schubert too was another composer who was bright, sparkling, clear and optimistic ... at least in this piece. The *Trout Quintet* based on the song was a special piece for her where all the instruments have their own voice and it was not just the first violin who was the star. She went on to describe the piano has having a very definite eddying about it.

MB: Eddying is the word, as it is about a trout in a stream. Going back to that time when you were young, you were also in the school choir and church choirs. Can you say something about your experience of singing in choirs?

Margaret: Yes ... At that stage we didn't have a piano and I suppose singing was my only way of making music. Singing in the car was really fun and a way of stopping the question 'Are we nearly there?'. Singing was very important both in primary and senior school. There were lots of choirs and chances to accompany on percussion, which I did ... I can still remember some of the words of the songs, for example, 'The chief defect of Henry King was chewing little bits of string'. We used to sing in competitions and I really do think that singing is an excellent way of involving people with music because there's no having to spend lots of money on an instrument. It's there, you have it already, and it's a great introduction to music and perhaps they can move on to appreciate other forms of music later.

MB: Yes, yes ... now the church choir that would have a different ambience about it?

Margaret: Mmn ... I don't remember that was quite as much fun ... but I do remember the carol singing ... and the memory of the tombs of the crusaders around and the one who had 14 children, it's quite set in my memory. I suppose all of that nurtured a historical interest.

MB: And an interest in architecture?

Margaret: Yes, that's definitely there.

MB: But it wasn't quite as much fun as singing about chewing bits of string?

Margaret: Definitely not!

I then asked Margaret if she had learned much from her piano lessons with the teacher with blue glasses and yellow hair. She recalled the piano lessons which were certainly different! She doesn't remember practising but she must have done because within two years she was playing quite complicated pieces, 'probably very badly' she adds, Then she moved to another teacher and she had to start again right at the beginning to correct her technique. But she recalls with affection her lessons with Madame Smith who was very exotic.

I noted that her father was an important figure for her musically and she remembered that they had a very good father/daughter relationship associated with music and she thinks that *The Trout* would always be one of her 'desert island discs' because of that. He had never had an opportunity to play an instrument and she remembers playing the piano aged about 12 and he remarking 'Oh play with some feeling!'. Margaret feels that he wanted to hear feeling in her music at a stage when she perhaps was a bit too young to express it in the particular piece of music. But Margaret's daughter Emily had piano lessons when young and Margaret says she was encouraged to sit next to her while she practised, and she thinks that was quite a good thing to do in that it showed she was interested, she could be encouraging and she could also help her to keep on track. The teacher was very sensitive to what a child of that age could take on board and was quite prepared to accept that one week she might be able to absorb lots in the lesson but at another lesson her concentration on the teaching might be only for five minutes. The rest of the time in that lesson would consist of piano games. I continued . . .

MB: That sounds very sensible . . . it sounds as if this teacher really listened to where the child was inside and tried to match the experience of music to this inner position. Thinking of matching music to an inner place, you write of music being very important for you therapeutically over the last eight years. Do you feel that you can say more about that perhaps?

Margaret: Yes . . . yes . . . I think it all ties in with the break-up of my marriage which was a time of great emotional upheaval. I had and have a lot of friends who were very supportive and I think I also used music as a prop . . . the music I listened to at this point in my life was quite safe and holding . . . I regard it as sort of musical counselling.

MB: Mmn . . .

Margaret: The sort of music I listened to was 'safe' . . . I didn't want to take in the experience of an emotional roller coaster . . . that was already happening in the rest of my life . . . I wanted something soothing that could hold me.

MB: What was the piece of music that was so important here?

Margaret: I think the Bach *Double Concerto for Two Violins and Orchestra* would be the main one.

MB: This is the piece we are going to talk about later but this was the special piece you listened to at that time?

Margaret: Yes . . . yes. It was a big contrast to what was happening in my life at that time and I think it was perhaps . . . me . . . taking the first steps . . . on a path . . . of my own . . . whether it was a literal path of being on my own or also a musical path . . . it was my own musical identity taking shape perhaps.

MB: Mmn . . . I wonder where you went after that musically? If Bach was the safe holding through the worst of the difficulties at that time . . . what did you listen to next on this path? What were you ready to take in next?

Margaret: Oh, what I think I really enjoyed then and enjoy doing now is losing myself in English twentieth century composers . . . not quite an experience of an emotional roller coaster but also not the degree of safety, should I say, of the Bach.

MB: Mmn . . . right.

Margaret: I particularly liked Delius' *The First Cuckoo in Spring* . . . and I can lose myself in the outside in my head . . . on my own . . . with my eyes closed . . . and smell the grass and hear that cuckoo which is so natural a sound compared with cuckoos in other pieces . . . it just seems so very natural.

MB: Yes . . . yes.

Margaret: And that's just me . . . I'm really an English country girl at heart.

MB: But there might be something else in there too . . . when you were listening to the Bach. It was soothing and holding . . . but in a sense there was no movement outward?

Margaret: Mmn . . .

MB: It was a soothing comforting experience?

Margaret: Mmn . . . yes.

MB: And there did seem to be something different happening within you when you listened to the Delius. You talk about moving outwards and it is almost as if you were daring to move outwards emotionally . . . but it may be that you are also saying . . . this is Englishness . . . this is me! Could it be that this is also something about who you are . . . and might this be the beginnings of a first step towards a newer sense of personal identity?

Margaret: Mmn . . . yes, I can say that it did feel more safe and was safe enough to step outside myself and listen to these new sounds from the outside world.

MB: It sounds as if perhaps you can also now take in other musical experiences because the Bach enveloped you at a time when you really needed this?

Margaret: Yes . . . yes.

MB: You can take in the sound of the cuckoo and you can 'smell the grass' . . . you can enjoy these things?

Margaret: Yes, indeed.

MB: It seems there is a kind of opening up happening . . . and it is very interesting?

Margaret: Mmn . . . there seems to be. I listen to a lot of Vaughan Williams too, his *Theme on Thomas Tallis* and the *Five Variants of 'Dives and Lazarus'*. I am really able to engage with this kind of music now.

MB: I wonder if alongside being able to engage with this different music you are also in some sense confirming who you are in your Englishness?

Margaret: Yes . . . yes . . . being confirmed . . . I understand that. I have become particularly fond of Benjamin Britten's music . . . and I think it's because one of my daughter's has been playing it a lot and the pieces I particularly like are unaccompanied.

MB: Unaccompanied . . . that's very interesting in itself.

Margaret: And it feels very free . . . no constraints . . . and there is more room just to play it differently . . . there is an exposure. You are very vulnerable unaccompanied but I like that in these pieces.

MB: If you were to draw a parallel from what you have just said about coming out of a dark period to a lighter place . . . its almost as if . . . there is a new sense of freedom around for you now . . . a different kind of life . . . would that feel right?

Margaret: Mmn . . . yes . . . I think so.

MB: You go on to write about enjoying the roller coaster of feelings in music now . . . that's going right out, isn't it. It sounds as if you are prepared . . .

At this point there was much laughter about the notion that Margaret was now prepared to give anything a go. 'In terms of music that is!', she added quickly.

MB: I wonder if you are able to trace some kind of journey here that is reflected through your changing preference in music?

Margaret: Yes . . . being serious for a moment, there has been a definite journey for me which I can see and have experienced. Music has accompanied me and I have felt the highs and the lows and I know I have lived with it and through it.

Margaret went on to talk about the memory of her children playing music at a concert and how she holds this in her mind. She described this as being almost better than a photograph because when she hears that piece of music she remembers them playing it. She added that it makes her feel very proud as a parent but wondered if she was a bit biased here. Her youngest daughter is also into jazz and she introduced Margaret to it.

Margaret felt that it must take a lot of courage to improvise in jazz and how incredible it is that someone can stand up with just a few chords in front of them and just 'make something utterly original out of them'. She really admires that they are prepared to stand up and be so exposed and take such a risk because it could all fall apart and they've got nothing to fall back on . "They've just got to give it a go and that's just great . . . ", she continued . . .

Margaret: It's a completely different atmosphere to any other music . . . I can't really enjoy jazz if there are all chairs in a row . . . I feel I need a glass in my hand! . . . Yes, I think it's wonderful.

MB: And it's very different from classical music which we have been talking about because that is generally all written down and very ordered and in that sense . . . very safe. You know what's round the corner . . . but you don't know what's round the corner at a jazz performance. It has that risk about it that classical music doesn't have.

Margaret: Exactly . . . there is a sense of humour in it too which I really enjoy.

MB: Music has become very important for you Margaret. Does it occupy some kind of a place inside you that you can visit when you want?

Margaret: I think this is a really difficult question for me to answer. I think it's just part of my soul. I think if you took it away . . . I would be very very unhappy . . . I think I could get quite depressed without music . . . it's part of my essence . . . I just love music . . . that's about all I can say.

MB: Perhaps Margaret we can go on to talk about the Bach *Double Concerto for Two Violins and Orchestra* which is your special choice of music.

Bach *Double Concerto for Two Violins and Orchestra in D minor*

The second movement of the *Double Concerto for Two Violins and Orchestra* is in ritornello form. A ritornello according to Frank Howes in *The Concerto*[1] is a kind of early rondo, the theme always returning but in different keys. This particular ritornello theme is said to enshrine the heart of the violin. It is passed with flowing elegance from one violin to the other.

MB: I wonder what your feelings are about this particular piece of music Margaret?

Margaret: I think the one word I would use above all others is serene . . . it is so beautiful and soothing as well . . . and the conversation between the two violins just passes seamlessly from one to the other. There is a sense of inevitability that it will just move on and continue to flow. I feel a sense of optimism because of that and it seems totally together in some way because of the accompaniment of the string orchestra. It feels very safe and I think this is why it was important for me in my life when my marriage was breaking down . . . I wasn't feeling safe then . . .

and this is also a pleasant conversation when my own conversations weren't pleasant . . . it was very protective . . . a way of holding me.

MB: Perhaps also enfolding you?

Margaret: Yes . . . it was protective . . . like a pair of wings coming around me . . . like a nice big duvet . . . warm and secure.

MB: Yes . . . that was very important for you then?

Margaret: Yes . . . .yes . . . I can't remember listening to it much before then, but I must have done. It was, however, just the right moment to find this piece in this way for me.

MB: It has this sublime quality of seemless flowing beauty as you say . . . a kind of endless quality about it . . . when it does end, what is your experience?

Margaret: I haven't thought about that before. It doesn't really bother me that it has ended . . . it doesn't feel final . . . I feel I could always come back to it.

MB: Yes, that's right.

Margaret: Some pieces of music feel very sad and the end feels very much that it *is* the end . . . the Elgar *Cello Concerto* would be an example of this . . . it is very tragic . . . and feels very sad.

MB: There is a real feeling of loss about it.

Margaret: Yes . . . while with the Bach there isn't that feeling of loss.

MB: I wonder if this is the note of optimism or hope you talked about earlier?

Margaret: Yes, yes.

MB: There is the feeling that it will be alright . . . here is another kind of response . . . here is the beautiful sound of another violin once more.

Margaret: There is no roller coaster there . . . it is so ordered and reliable. Even though it has ended and been taken away from you . . . you can just smoothly move on.

MB: I wonder if there is a sense in which there is always music going on in the world although we don't hear it. It is out there in the ether . . . this 'to and fro' flow in sound vibrations is going on . . . and this piece of music seems to resonate with this idea?

Margaret: Yes.

MB: And there is nothing jarring. It is really interesting that it is all strings . . . if there was another instrument there I wonder what it would feel like?

Margaret: It would feel as if it was a distraction from the uncomplicated simplicity and feeling of wholeness . . . if there was an oboe there it would seem totally inappropriate.

MB: And perhaps it would be saying 'Look at me'?

Margaret: Yes it would . . . and that's not what this piece is about. It is balanced and ordered and it is right that it is strings only . . . to me it is as near perfection as one can get in music.

MB: Thank you very much Margaret.

References

1 Howes F (1968) Johann Sebastian Bach. In: R Hill (ed.) *The Concerto*. Penguin Books, Harmondsworth, p. 19.

CHAPTER 11

Interview with
The Reverend Reg Dean

Reg was 100 years old on 4 November 2002 and is still singing in the choir, although he did not go with them to the South of France as he had planned. He recently gave Mary North his recipe for a long life – a sound faith, friends and family to love, involvement in music and becoming a vegetarian. (Mary North very kindly facilitated this interview.)

Reg's writing

**[Reg dictated his account of his experiences of music to Mary North –
8 January 2003]**

When I listen to music I get a feeling, an emotion which I don't get otherwise. It's different from the emotions I feel with people or with reading. It's particularly associated with music. It's hard to say any more about it, but it's different from the joy you get from 'elevated thought' as I think Wordsworth puts it in *Tintern Abbey*. It is something deep. There is something in me which requires satisfaction, which is not satisfied by something airy and light, but is more tragic. I do not think it is to do with the approach of death for it has been so for a long time.

My musical education was sadly neglected and was not awakened until middle age. I always enjoyed singing though, tuneful songs and melodies. I deeply deplore that they have given way to punk rock which I find an anguished shouting, not melodious singing, but it is made attractive to young people by lighting effects and attractive presentation.

My musical education, if you can call it that, was awakened in India about 1938. I suddenly felt the need to hear instrumental music in concert. I bought a gramophone and began to buy 78 rpm records. I remember especially enjoying Beethoven's *Seventh Symphony*. I had a need which was connected with a deepening religious thought and later a connection developed between music and words. I later made experiments of reading within a musical context, not accompaniment as such, but with music. I was writing lots of poems at this same time of religious exploration.

The experience of listening to music then brought a certain satisfaction. It supplied something which was lacking in my awareness of life and art and spiritual experience. I'm afraid my training as a priest was rather cerebral. But since those days I have always connected thought and feeling very closely. I feel my 'composition', emotional, mental and spiritual has never been as fully integrated as I would have wished. Music helps me towards this end. Music for me initially did not have a relational context but came as a development of religious feeling. For example, about this time around 1940, the French horn became very eloquent to me because of its tone. It figures in Grieg's *Piano Concerto* which is one of my favourite pieces, but my really favourite pieces of music are Rachmaninov's *Second Piano Concerto* and Tchaikovsky's *Sixth Symphony*.

My experience of music has not changed in itself but has come to play an increasingly large part in my mental and spiritual experience. However, I think in the tokens of experience, words mean more than anything else to me, and this happened before my sight began to fail. But I have always been associated with male voice choirs and still sing in one. My father was in a male voice choir and I first heard this choir when I was aged 15 or so at Newcastle-under-Lyme and was deeply impressed by the harmonies. A friend of my father was a conductor and composer, and he wrote a setting of *Hereward the Wake*. I've sung in male voice choirs most of my adult life and listened a lot too. The choir is very important to me – the timbre of male voices and the harmonies are just short of miraculous and I am, perhaps, part of that lovely sound. I have always felt that the human voice is the most wonderful of musical instruments. My favourite singer used to be Peter Dawson, a baritone who sang mainly ballads. I'm deeply impressed too by Gilbert and Sullivan, partly because they are witty. Big band and jazz, however, seem to be too superficial and not soul-searching. If there is heaven it must be the musical experience of singing.

I listen to music at any time, at all times! If I couldn't it would be like the sunshine taken out of the day; the brilliance would be missing. I wrote a poem entitled *Music*, in India about 1940. It is inspired by a pianist who introduced me to All India Radio. She was a friend and music teacher and we broadcast together, me singing ballads with her accompanying.

Music – **The Reverend Reg Dean**

Under the night sky, glimmering coldly
Shines a dream of you.
Into the wide light fierce at noontime
Living all day through.

Naught in all this changing life scene
Shadows the peace I know,
If beyond the claims of darkness
Measures of rapture grow.

Stay oh stay sublimest of Muses
Whilst soft voices fall:
Earth is afire with echoes of heaven,
Quickening to thy call.

Lovely hands the strains awaken
Tuning each trembling string,
Beauty to thy themes imparting
Richly as they sing.

Through the steep resounding heavens
Let your music rise,
Shed its rare and burning splendour
Down the waiting skies.

This I think shows that music had evidently become a living thing with me. Players and singers *are* associated with the art itself.

Conversation with Reg

MB: Reg, in your writing you say that music occupies a place in your mind which is special and which invites a sense of deep longing. Can you say something more about this?

Reg: Yes ... this place is like a rose on my 'peace' rose bush in my garden. This beautiful flower has a certain shape which develops as it blooms. First there is a tight bud and then there is a gradual opening and then the delicate pink and yellow and white colours appear in the full blown rose. This for me is like the evolution of my experience in appreciating the musician's art, an unfolding of beauty.

MB: So music for you is like this rose opening up revealing ever more beauty. This would describe that place of music for you in your heart?

Reg: I know this beauty is there in the world but I am not fully aware of it at all times. But I become aware of it through my experience of music ... but my musical education was neglected I'm afraid.

MB: Tell me about that Reg.

Reg: I suppose it really began for me in my middle age in India around 1938 ... it was Beethoven's *Seventh Symphony* which was the 'awakening'.

MB: An awakening of what Reg?

Reg: Not a causal awakening . . . it was an accompanying awakening to a deeper layer of religious experience which enveloped me at that time. Music came with it not as a result of it.

MB: You were opening up like the rose. Tell me about that time Reg.

Reg: I had begun a new ministry of work in Bombay as minister of a church and I was meeting my congregation and making friends, etc., but I became aware of the need for a fuller expression of the thought and feeling that religious experience brings. I also became acquainted with the Oxford Movement Group and the Moral Rearmament Movement which opened up doors for me that hitherto had been closed on emotion. I had only considered problems of life intellectually until then. It was as if I had passed out from the intellectual room in my mind into the emotional room carrying with me a trail of the intellectual as well.

MB: What was it Reg that was behind this shift from the intellectual room into the emotional room?

Reg: I think it was seeing the needs of the people and the goodness of people amidst the awful poverty around me . . . the weight and power of that experience brought about that shift which engaged my emotions in a new way. So much so that I spoke to the Bishop and tried to outline a scheme of employment for the poor. This was a way of social action in a practical way. But the Bishop answered to the effect that this was a pipe dream and "Did I not have something more detailed in mind?" I then met my friend David Creed. He was an Eurasian and an officer in Eurasian society in Bombay and we shared this concern. They were very difficult days for unemployment. It was just after the world depression, the effects still lingered. We couldn't do much but I did find work for several young men and I remember one became a verger at the Anglican Church . . . and that had not a lot to do with the Bishop . . . but it was so long ago it has passed into the vague relics of memory.

MB: You also include your fine poem of that time inspired by your friendship with a pianist in 1940.

At this point Reg began to remember how he became friendly with the church secretary Philip Harper and his wife Beryl who lived in Matunga. Nearby lived Agnes Barrett who used to play the piano and give recitals on All India Radio. Reg was invited to sing ballads with Agnes accompanying and they used to broadcast these recitals which included Masefield's *Sea Songs* and 'rollicking songs' like the *Bold Bad Banderillero*. He remembered that Agnes taught him a lot about music and as he says 'enhanced his appreciation of it'. We returned to our conversation to include his reflections on music and words.

MB: Reg, you wrote about your developing connection between music and words. Can you say something about this?

Reg: Well I used to feel that words were . . . things. But they were not just ciphers. I realised that they were an expression of thought in a material way and so they were a medium of sound. I have always loved the sound of words, the onomato-poeia of words, and I began to connect them with musical sound, and I would further combine them in my thought and experience and would sit down and develop my platform recitals – performances of poetry or prose readings with a musical accompaniment. I used to memorise and recite stories by O'Henry for example, or Browning's *Pied Piper of Hamelin* or Shakespeare's Hamlet soliloquy and I spoke these to a musical background.

MB: Can you give me an example of one with a musical background?

Reg: Well, yes . . . I spoke Milton's *Paradise Lost* to Beethoven's *Fifth Symphony*, the first movement. I was indeed interested in music and words and I was a founder member of the Bombay Light Opera Company and used to sing parts in their per-formances. I feel that words themselves are musical and they are almost asking for musical notes to be associated with them.

[Reg then recalled, in an aside, that he was at one time invited to be part of the audition/examination board for the Guildhall School of Music and Drama in London.]

MB: Are there particular words now that come to mind as you reflect on this?

Reg: Yes, the words of *Tintern Abbey* by Wordsworth are particularly musical.

Tintern Abbey

. . . . 'For I have learned
To look on nature, not as in the hour
Of thoughtless youth; but in hearing often-times
The still sad music of humanity,
Nor harsh nor grating, though of ample power
To chasten and subdue. And I have felt
A presence that disturbs me with the joy
Of elevated thoughts; a sense sublime
Of something far more deeply interfused,
Whose dwelling is the light of setting suns,
And the round ocean and the living air,
And the blue sky, and in the mind of man:
A motion and a spirit, that impels
All thinking things, all objects of all thought,
And rolls through all things.'

MB: This seems to have a very special meaning for you, this passage?

Reg: Yes, indeed, I can see through the clouds of problematic evil that make nature so confused and confusing and admire it and think how beautiful it is;

but I am aware at the same time of the millions of tragedies that are going on underneath its surface. It is this beauty on one side and tragedy on the other ... I have no answer to it ... but the Christian experience is a relief from it.

MB: Reg ... you say in your writing that your training as a priest was a rather cerebral experience?

Reg: Yes, I was trained as an Anglican priest. The college, St Augustine's, was a very beautiful place, beautiful buildings, beautiful quadrangle and next door to the Canterbury Hospital. This was also, by the way, part of my youthful experience because the senior surgeon used to invite students from the college to witness operations and I was one of those invited. I also used to help in the outpatients department. It was all part of our development.

MB: Yes indeed ... your training for the priesthood.

Reg: On the religious side I must say I tended to be content with the theological questions rather than the experiential side of life and I used to be one of those who examined articles of religion and faith to find out what they meant, what the words meant – very cerebral! And I did rather thrive on the idea that our faith had been laid down in the past and was unchangeable. I felt reason had to govern the enquiry and I spent years asking questions about the meaning of faith, the faith I was supposed to profess! ... I'm embarrassed about that now!

MB: You smile about that now Reg. I wonder what that's about?

Reg: Yes ... I rather succeeded in what I was doing, this cerebral enquiry, and did very well in my exams. But now I think my exams were really a means of expressing in thought the experiences I had in feeling, and until I began to marry these aspects together I was not connected up in the most important way.

MB: And that's the important picture we first have of you in India, in Bombay, when thought and feeling merged within you. And this enabled you to set up your ideas of work for the poor, your social action. You write, music was important for you at that time in Bombay and I know you said that this experience of music wasn't causal to any change that followed, but could it be thought of as a new pathway linking thought and feeling perhaps ... a pathway accompanying you on your life journey?

Reg: Yes, it was. It's about experiencing the new in being human. 'In my father's house there are many mansions', many ways of living the spiritual life ... I am in a mansion, as I was then ... and I explore by opening doors to beauty in all its forms ... the furniture may be different in each room and the sounds may be different but I am able to experience life in its various aspects and not be rigid.

MB: And that for you would be a spiritual quest and your 'awakening' accompanied by music was and is an important aspect here. You do say, however, that words mean more than anything else to you. Could you say a bit more about that?

Reg: The combination of words we use, the way that we express ourselves in words and the feelings we have, can be done gracefully, sometimes flatly, sometimes with more meaning. It is how we express who we are in communication that is important.

MB: That's very interesting and it has to do with intonation, *how* we say the words. But how do we bring people in here? When you are describing this, words sound as if they are on the page. How do we begin to talk about persons in this?

Reg: I don't live in the abstract . . . I live in reality and persons mean more to me than abstract thoughts and opinions. And, however I may deplore the opinions of my friends, I regard them as persons whom I can like and love. I've always been inclined to look for the best in people not the worst. There are, of course, some people whose company you can't enjoy for more than half-an-hour before you'll hear something to the discredit of somebody else . . . that disturbs me. But if we take the words of Jesus and the words of Liturgy in Church, they carry so much affirmation of what it is to be a human being. That is what has helped build my religious life. The affirmation which these words express . . . that is what is important . . . doubts are always with me but you can affirm a feeling or a belief without having to take it to pieces which is what I used to try to do.

MB: And that is what draws you to the person of Jesus?

Reg: As I once said . . . "If it wasn't for the person of Jesus I would be an atheist". It is to do with the person because I can't become reconciled to the natural order of the world with all its cruelty and which is supposed to have been created by a loving God.

MB: And it is the person of Jesus speaking these words of affirmation?

Reg: He absorbed all the evil that assailed him and converted it.

MB: Yes . . . you say that you began to link words with music long before your sight began to fail. When did you begin to lose your sight Reg?

Reg: I was registered blind five years ago but my sight began to fail before that although it wasn't until I was 50 I began to wear glasses.

Reg went on to say that he could read distinctly until he was about 70 and it was then that he began to realise that he was having trouble reading in church and some of the words were becoming blurred. He added mischievously that he had to substitute some of his own then. But 10 years ago when he was 90 he began to definitely feel that blindness was coming on and five years later he was registered blind. He says, however, that he still has some peripheral vision. We moved on to talk about the fact that he still sings in a choir.

MB: You write about choirs Reg, and how important that singing in a choir is for you?

Reg: Yes . . . it brings with it this special experience of being part of a larger lovely sound because of the harmony. And the harmony brings us together; and the members of the choir, I know, are working together, thinking together and enjoying together . . . they are more like a band of brothers rather than a group of singers only.

At this point Reg reminded me that he had to go on to a choir rehearsal that evening after our interview. He sings bass in the choir, The Dalesmen Male Voice Choir, and he is going to France with the choir, to Bergerac at the end of May. He also mentioned that as well as being a choir member he is its President.

MB: You finish you writing Reg, by saying that music is a living thing for you to do with persons . . . can you say a bit more about that?

Reg: Yes, yes it's embodied in persons . . . it's performed by persons. I'm afraid the idea of writing music is way beyond anything I can comprehend . . . but making music, as in singing, I can understand.

MB: You write that if there is a heaven it must be the musical experience of singing?

Reg: Yes . . . I think of singing filling the air of heaven . . . the air *ring* . . . *ing* with sound . . . not perpetual sound of course . . . that I think would detract from the beauty of the experience.

MB: Yes . . . to really appreciate sound you have to have silence?

Reg: Yes . . . but I think of the air *ring* . . . *ing*!

MB: Perhaps Reg, we can turn to your chosen music of Rachmaninov.

Rachmaninov's *Second Piano Concerto in C# minor* – the second movement

---

This concerto's first performance was in 1901 and, although written at the beginning of the twentieth century, the style of writing in this concerto belongs to the late romantic school of the previous century.

In the music there is a strong sense of drama allied to powerful lyrical melodic writing. John Culshaw in *The Concerto*[1] describes the Rachmaninov concertos as being 'dominated by the more immediate of the darker emotions'.[1] It was written shortly after Rachmaninov had recovered from a mental breakdown.

MB: This second movement Reg, comes after the drama of the first movement. What do you feel about this short movement?

Reg: There is something hauntingly beautiful about the intervals of the melody.

MB: The distances between the flow of the notes and the fall of the phrase.

Reg: They seem to carry with them a sadness . . . a plaintive sound which in the hands of a musician becomes a thing of beauty . . . and the conversation between the different instruments, the woodwind and the piano and the strings is a kind of interfused beauty.

MB: They combine together, converse . . . in this beautiful sound.

Reg: It is an important part of life I think to combine together in an enterprise or an exploration.

MB: Music here would be symbolic of this perhaps, this coming together to form something beautiful?

Reg: But there is more . . . I love scintillating conversation and I enjoy it but there is something beyond this as well. 'That still sad music of humanity' flowing beneath it, bearing it up. The joy and the rollicking jokes are a welcome part of life, but not the essence of life.

MB: At the beginning of your writing, Reg, you talk of music as having a tragic depth to it. You write . . . 'It is something deep . . . there is something deep in me that is not satisfied with the airy and light'.

Reg: Yes . . . I think that the essence of life as we know it here on earth is a tragedy . . . it may be great to experience rollicking joy and scintillating conversation, but there is a tragic underflow.

MB: And this second movement of the Rachmaninov *Second Piano Concerto* . . .

Reg: Carries this feeling and thought.

MB: Going back to the image of the rose unfolding Reg, where is this sense of tragedy here?

Reg: Well I don't think it is approaching death because I have lived with that too long and considered that many times. Blake refers to it in 'O rose thou art sick, the invisible worm' . . . the tragedy at the heart of beauty . . . the bitter sweetness of life.

MB: Thank you Reg.

The Sick Rose – **William Blake**

O rose thou art sick!
The invisible worm
That flies in the night
In the howling storm,

Has found out thy bed
Of crimson joy,
And his dark secret love
Does thy life destroy.

This poem has been set to music by Benjamin Britten in the *Serenade for Tenor, Horn and Strings*.

References

1 Culshaw J (1968) Sergei Rachmaninov and Nicholas Medtner. In: *The Concerto*. R Hill (ed.) Penguin Books, Harmondsworth, p. 290.

CHAPTER 12

Interview with Susan McGinness

Susan had a long career as a professional flautist playing with orchestras and chamber groups. She is now a counsellor working with young people in Scotland.

Susan's writing

I suppose the great irony of my life is that, having lived and breathed music from the age of five, and even earlier, I rarely listen to it now. I think this is not because it has come to mean so little to me, but because it still means so much.

My earliest memory of music is hearing my father's recording of the Bach/Vivaldi harpsichord concertos as a very small child, lying awake in the dark after having been put to bed. While I was ultimately the only professional musician in the family, ours was a musical household; my father played the double bass in a doctor's jazz band, my sister played the piano (more out of duty and expectation, probably, than real interest) and my mother loved the great operatic voices of Joan Sutherland, Renata Tebaldi and Franco Corelli.

I think I was a natural musician. When I was three or four years old I begged to have piano lessons like my big sister. They didn't last long because my attention span was too short at that age, but I amazed my mother at a parents' evening at school by marching out on stage and playing the piece my sister had been studying for her piano lesson that week which I had learned by ear. At the age of five, my best friend Sandy, who already played the violin, took up the flute. I know now that the flute was never my voice (I should have been a cellist or perhaps a horn player), but I knew nothing much about the other options then and wanted to be like Sandy, so I became a flautist. We made music together until her family moved away when we were 12. It was around that time that I think I began to practise because I wanted to, rather than being reminded by my mother. That was also when I metamorphosed from a confident, friendly child into an introverted and self-conscious adolescent, although the process had already begun a year earlier when I developed an eating disorder which was to be part of my life for almost 30 years.

Yet inside that starved and withdrawn teenager was a great passion for which I had no words, but which responded with tremendous intensity to *music*, both as I played it and listened to it. It was the big nineteenth century romantics that spoke for me – Bruckner's *Ninth Symphony*, Brahms' *Second Symphony*, Rachmaninoff, Wagner. By this time I was principle flute in a prestigious youth orchestra and was playing many of the great orchestral works for the first time. I will never forget our initial rehearsal of Elsa's Procession to the Cathedral, from *Lohengrin*. I now recognise my response to it as an almost sexual one but then could barely find words to describe it although I tried, only to be hugely embarrassed when my parents discovered what I had secretly written.

I had a great talent but was never very happy as a concerto soloist. Once, when I was 15 or 16, I happened to be hanging around waiting for a rehearsal to start while auditions for a solo prize were going on so I did an audition for a lark and, to my horror, promptly won it playing *Syrinx* by Debussy. Looking back now, I can see how astounding it must have been for such a big, warm, erotic performance to have come from such a non-descript, mousey stick as I was then. As a counsellor who works with young people, I am incredibly angry now that no-one ever asked me what was wrong, or did anything to acknowledge my desperate – and very visible – unhappiness other than to make me keep a food diary for a week. I think that music literally saved my life. When I was playing, when I was sitting in the middle of an orchestra, I could soar, I could be noticed; it didn't matter what I looked like or what was going on at home, and the monstrous conspiracy of silence that surrounded it all.

Over the following years I had an ambivalent relationship with music. I quit playing, then would practise my heart out, get a job and then quit again. As my world grew, as I discovered my physical and intellectual self, I had other means of expression that had previously been limited only to the flute, although music remained the deepest and most genuine connection to who I was. In fact, it wasn't until fairly late in my career when a colleague in the orchestra I was playing in at the time took me aside and had a word with me about my very emotional response to being told I would not be playing in the Strauss *Serenade for Wind*, that I began to see music more as a job than as an extension of myself. This visceral approach to music made me an exceptionally expressive and communicative performer, but was a liability to me when it came to surviving in the cut-throat world of professional classical music.

Perhaps the epitome of what music meant to me as a performer is implicit in the fact that I chose to play at my mother's funeral rather than to be in the congregation. I decided to play Gounod's *O Divine Redeemer*, one of her favourites. While I chose it for its beautiful melody, it wasn't until just before the service that I read the words, which turned out to be so apt for my mother's life, and her death by suicide. While people seem amazed that I could play at her funeral, I can't see how I could have done anything else; my playing said everything for me, as it always did.

When I think about my relationship with music now, I realise that I do much the same thing, although I am no longer playing – I use it to express, or to connect with, strong feelings. I rarely listen just for pleasure, and never as background. For the first few years after I stopped playing I found I could not bear to hear music or see it performed. My grief at having to give it up is buried deeper now, and when I choose a particular CD to match my mood, I can access that same connection, those same intense emotions I felt all those years ago as a child full of passions

I could only harness through music. Now, with the benefit of a great deal of my own life and, I guess, through 10 years of being a therapist, and experiencing the heights and depths of the human condition on a larger scale, the difference is that I can recognise what the music is saying to me rather than using it as a voice for myself to speak to others.

Conversation with Susan

MB: Susan, you say that you rarely listen to music now because it means so much to you. You may want to say more later but do you feel you can say something now?

Susan: Ah . . . I think it's . . . so much a part of me and I think of myself as a musician even though I no longer perform. In my soul I am a musician and I think there is something about the disharmony in myself about feeling that and not doing it. That is something quite painful and so I don't listen to music much. Anything that reminds me . . . is a grief. And I think this was the case even when I was playing . . . I value silence. I love silence . . . the kind of silence you get on the top of a mountain that's so absolute you can feel it.

MB: Yes . . . yes.

Susan: That kind of silence is alive and I crave it . . . so I'm not somebody who wants much going on soundwise. If I want to listen to music I choose it. I almost never have the radio on in the background . . . never! I think it's the pain in it I don't want to experience .

MB: It's the pain in the music you are talking about?

Susan: Yes . . . mmn . . . yes.

MB: You say that you should have been a cellist Susan or a horn player. Could you say a bit more about your preference for these instruments?

Susan: It's the timbre in the sound they make. I started playing the flute when I was five and it has these twiddly sounds and squeaks and the person I grew into from that five-year-old wanted to play Beethoven quartets. I needed something to sink my teeth into . . . a richer sound . . . an alto sound. My singing voice is an alto. I'm really not a flute player and I think that's something to do with a kind of love/hate affair I have with the instrument. I would play and then quit and then play and quit . . . I never really felt it was my voice.

MB: Yes . . . you say that in your writing.

Susan: And the cello repertoire is wonderful . . . those concertos!

MB: Yes, the whole range of music . . . I'm wondering if there is a richness in the cello that you just can't hear in the flute?

Susan: Yes that's right . . . and string quartets are the ultimate music aren't they?

MB: What is it Susan about string quartets that is so supreme . . . it seems to be the highest musical experience for you?

Susan: It reduces and intensifies at the same time . . . and there is also something about playing in a small ensemble. Ah . . . If you watch the great quartets they play as one . . . and the eye contact is wonderful. I think there is nothing better than playing in small groups. You have a different kind of relationship with them than you have with an orchestra which is another kind of big thrill. There is still an intimacy there but at another level. You are part of something which is much bigger than you. You have more of a sense of your own voice in a string quartet. But it is marvellous to be in the middle of Beethoven's *Ninth Symphony* . . . you feel you are part of something outside yourself. You feel that playing in the quartet as well, but there is something special too about being part of this huge community of players.

Susan went on to describe being a musical child in a musical family and therefore exposed to a wide range of music from Bach to opera to jazz. She recalled in particular the Bach-Vivaldi harpsichord concertos from that time. Her memory was of her being in bed and hearing this music. Her father would play a recording of this piece. She also remembered opera recordings her mother played. I asked her what she remembered in particular about the Bach-Vivaldi recording.

Susan: It had such vitality, I want to dance to it now!! And the sound of four harpsichords and string orchestra . . . it's such a great sound. Wow! . . . I find it difficult to attach this to an exact memory. It was just there as an early experience.

MB: At the age of 12 you lost your best friend Sandy who was also a flautist. Are you able to say a bit about that time. Sandy leaving must have been a real sadness for you then?

Susan: It was. It was a strange time to lose a best friend. That's the time when you really want your best friends around you and I think I withdrew a bit as a result. I went to visit her in North Carolina and we still have a strong connection today. We speak every birthday on the telephone.

MB: I'm thinking about what happened to you after she left. At 12 it is hard to lose your best friend. Did you talk about it to anyone?

Susan: No . . . I never talked about anything to anybody,

MB: You played the flute. Perhaps you put all this into music?

Susan: Possibly . . . but I didn't realise that at the time. I just got on with it and I am not sure things would have been all that different if she had stayed. This was the time when I was in junior high school and I remember it was very important how you looked. I had big thick glasses and I was no great beauty and by that time I had begun to lose a lot of weight. So I was very skinny and ugly with big glasses . . . so it was not a very easy time . . . very painful.

MB: Around that time you write that you changed from practising because you were told to by your mother, to practising because you wanted to.

Susan: I don't quite know what the reason for that was. Perhaps it was because I realised I was very different from my peers. Different because I was not particularly attractive and I was also fairly bright. I was one of those 'geeks'. You know . . . the class 'geek' . . . and so music was somewhere where it didn't matter how I looked. It was a world in which I could shine!

MB: Yes . . . you could excel here.

Susan: Also I felt accepted for myself in music . . . when I went to rehearsals in the orchestra and would horse around with everyone, people liked me. It was my world. I didn't feel this in early middle school. When I went to a school for children of higher IQ it was better there. Then I started to practise for myself. It was as if I was grabbing on to something that was me . . . where what I looked like didn't matter.

MB: And what you grabbed at was in music?

Susan: Yes . . . yes. I could still feel awkward generally but when I played at rehearsal or performance . . . that was great.

MB: You remind me Susan of a fish out of water. When it's out of water it's awkward and if you put it back in water it swims beautifully.

Susan: But if I had been beautiful then . . . who knows what would have happened.

MB: You write Susan that you developed an eating disorder . . . are you able to say something about this?

Susan went on to describe how she thought that this eating disorder came from her family situation. Her mother was addicted to prescribed drugs and she was ill a lot of the time with migraine headaches. Susan thought a lot of it was psychosomatic and also her mother suffered from postnatal depression after Susan was born. She was never diagnosed or treated – the medication was all for the migraines and other things and she never recovered from this. In the 1950s this was not discussed much, according to Susan. Her mother was ill for most of Susan's life and she says she grew up feeling abandoned in the sense that her mother was not there for her most of the time. She notes that there was something about engagement and attachment between her mother and her which just couldn't happen because her mother was ill and not emotionally available for her.

Also the relationship between her mother and father was very poor. He would leave the house at 7 o'clock in the morning so he was absent as well. Susan recalled that there were lots of family stories about what she did as a child and all of them were because she was on her own with no one looking after her. I asked if there was one story she could remember in particular.

Susan: Well there was the one when the local farmer used to deliver an order of bacon, eggs, butter, etc. which my mother had ordered. As usual I was on my own when he made the delivery and he left it in the sitting room. When my mother came down eventually, I had spread the butter into the sofa and draped the bacon over the back ... I was about four or five ... and there are a number of such stories.

Susan then remembered another particular instance of feeling very alone. This time it was about the fear of an absent father.

Susan: I can remember at a very young age being curled up on the floor in my bedroom which was above the kitchen and trying to hear what my parents were fighting about.

MB: That's really hard.

Susan: And thinking ... oh ... is it about me or my dad? ... because I was afraid he was going to leave ... and my father was the *one* ... he was it! He was the one the sun shone from for me.

MB: The anchor in your family?

Susan: Even though I didn't see much of him ... he was a respected hospital doctor ... he was the one I really connected with and so I had a great fear that he would leave I think ... and when I would hear 'I'm only staying here because of the children' ... I think the seeds were sown for a high level of anxiety in me.

Susan went on to recall the Berlin and the Cuban crises. Her father was in the reserve medical corps and very committed. She remembers the terror she experienced that he might be called up at any time during that period. She was 11 then and links this with the start of her eating disorder. She remembers listening to the radio for news about the crises and being terrified. She recalls that this depth of fear is still with her and that's why she is afraid of flying and how she is sometimes terrified that something awful is going to happen in some form or other. We returned to her weight loss and how no one seemed to notice.

MB: You say that when you were 11 you started losing weight?

Susan: I starved myself ... for years ... and nobody said 'What's wrong?'. My father made me write down everything I ate for a week and that was all the acknowledgement I got that I was doing this to myself ... that was it. That makes me angry ... angry to this day.

MB: It was a complete taboo?

Susan: It is a taboo in families anyway ... I work a lot with young people with eating disorders ... and I understand this ... it's a big secret And back then in 1961 there was nothing in the popular magazines about it as there is now ... so I proceeded to starve myself for many years and then it became a binge/starve kind of thing. I had a disordered relationship with food up until I was about 40 really.

MB: What do you understand the root of this to have been here?

Susan: I think it was about control. I couldn't control my mother in terms of what I needed from her and I couldn't control whether my father would leave or not and possibly be killed in a war.

MB: You would survive if you could control what you took in?

Susan: Well . . . you *are* surviving if you can control this . . . you're surviving your life . . . because nothing else might survive. I'd come home to a mother who half the time would be unconscious on the floor from an overdose of drugs . . . so life was chaotic. But in and through all of this I had my music and I could envelop myself in that. It didn't matter . . . nothing else mattered . . . when I was playing music I was high as a kite . . . it saved my life . . . it really did.

MB: It is interesting that music has this real feeling of safety for some people?

Susan: It wasn't only that. It was how I could get it all out . . . all those feelings. Music allowed me to feel on all levels, from passion to spiritual feelings like those I wrote about in Elsa's procession. I could feel those feelings and I felt connected up.

MB: This seems quite important that from this little child who felt not connected up you could begin to feel more connected up later in life through music?

Susan: It allowed me to express those feelings inside me and also to connect up with the bigger world . . . by this bigger world I think I mean a kind of spiritual place. I felt I tapped into something.

MB: You could be yourself in music and be accepted by other people?

Susan: Yes . . . and I was never conscious of how I looked when I was playing . . . that was still the incongruent bit of me. I wasn't very glamourous, but boy!, I was a passionate, passionate girl and clearly music allowed me to express all of this.

MB: You write that you were never very comfortable as a soloist as time went on?

Susan: Yes, I began to have a horror of actually having to perform a piece in front of an audience by myself.

Staying with this feeling of aloneness, Susan continued to recall occasions when she had to perform as a soloist and was then so self-conscious. She never thought that this might change one day. There didn't seem to be anyone around to encourage her in this way. In this sense she has always felt alone in her life.

She has had, as she says, several relationships in her life but lives on her own and has done so for years and puts it down to the fact that from birth she has had this sense of being on her own. Susan then continued . . .

Susan: And maybe some of those kinds of feelings of being essentially on my own were there in utero for me. Certainly after I was born and gradually able to think I assumed I was on my own.

MB: Somewhere, somehow you knew about this?

Susan: And through adolescence, when most people are more self-aware, I knew sharply I was on my own.

MB: It stays with you doesn't it?

There is current research in neuroscience which explores the sense of aloneness of the infant in utero and how this persists if the mother continues to suffer
from depression.[1]

Then this part of the conversation about feeling alone and still having to perform in front of an audience on a big occasion brought Susan to talking about an
incident just before her last public performance as a musician playing in the
Queen Elizabeth Hall in 1992. It was with the group Hausmusik which was and
is as she says a 'Rolls Royce' chamber group which she founded in 1986, and as
she put it, just 'forgot' to mention it in her writing!

Susan then began to tell me about the incident concerning her last performance at the Queen Elizabeth Hall.

Susan: I was very very nervous about this concert. I took myself to Cornwall and
practised for a week before the concert. I was terrified . . . and then I had a great
revelation that the things that I had done since my mother had died in 1978,
teaching, writing, for example, I had done with great confidence and the music I
had played from an early age was in some way associated with her in that I had no
confidence in my playing *now*.

It seemed that no matter how brilliantly I played the flute at school I could
never get that thing from her that I needed. I was all the time searching for that
something in the playing of my music.

But following on from that revelation and a few days before the concert at the
Queen Elizabeth Hall I visited a Jungian therapist. I said I had just understood this
and didn't know what to do with all of what this might mean. It was such a huge
understanding for me. She said she thought that I might be right . . . but there
wasn't much time before the concert to do a great deal of work on my terror and
fear. She then suggested a good acupuncturist who might be able to help in the
immediate instance.

I visited the acupuncturist and I'm phobic about needles. She started off by
taking my pulses and then she said that, yes, there was definitely someone else
in there and said she would try to get that someone out. This was frightening for
me and I had the most awful fear that I was going to die. I felt as if I was losing
myself in some way. The acupuncturist was saying 'Keep your eyes open or I will
lose you'. I was frightened out of my wits because I didn't know what was happening . . . but when it was over and I came to . . . I felt newborn in a sense. I had to
take a cab and I was so poor in those days I never took cabs, but I felt I couldn't
go out in the outside world I felt so new . . . new and raw and sort of unpeeled . . .
it was an extraordinary sensation. The concert went fine!

MB: That's a remarkable story.

Susan: I don't know if I'm completely purged yet of all of what was in there . . . but
something came out.

MB: Something came out and you were freed up in some way?

Susan: I was freed up of something . . . and the tragedy is that I didn't realise this
until my very last performance . . . but there you go.

MB: So how about this last performance . . . how was it that it was your last performance?

Susan: Oh, because I had just applied and become accepted to train as a counsellor in Scotland.

MB: But in 1992 you found this real feeling of freedom for you to be you . . . yet you decided not to continue with music with this new freedom?

Susan: Oh . . . there were also all sorts of practical outside reasons like problems with work permits and visas . . . my musical career in England was dogged with difficult problems. There was also a kind of closed shop mentality in the flute playing world, one person decided who was going to play and who wasn't. There was a lot of political wrangling in the business side of orchestral flute playing.

MB: You write very movingly about playing the flute at your mother's funeral. You were saying 'goodbye' to her?

Susan: That was in 1978. I expect I was saying something of a 'goodbye' . . . and it was also my way of coping with the funeral. Everybody blamed me and my father for her death . . . and none of my mother's family or friends spoke to me at the funeral. It was a difficult time and if there were strong feelings around I wanted to be playing. Also I didn't know what to do and I wanted to contribute something but I didn't want to speak. I think in some way I also wanted to absent myself from the funeral so I was up in the choir loft with a dear friend who was an organist and very supportive. I could just be there with my music and a supportive friend and somehow get through the funeral that way.

MB: Yes . . . it was your way of getting through this difficult time?

Susan: It *was* a 'goodbye' to her . . . and I played one of her favourite pieces *O Divine Redeemer* . . . she loved that piece. That was something that harked back to those early years when she played a lot of vocal music.

After a short time to give some space before continuing, we returned to talking about Susan's present relationship with music.

Susan: My relationship with music now isn't one of me *making* music actively, which was a way of using music to express myself whilst also escaping from the unpleasant stuff of living. Now that I don't have the emotional investment in music in that it had to be my only voice . . . I can now hear it!!

MB: What is it saying to you?

Susan: When I listen to the last works of the great composers like Beethoven quartets, there is something in their writing that transcends . . . I listen to them for comfort. I have a great fear of dying . . . because there is so much that I want to do and it's not fair that I am 53. When I listen to the Bach cantatas and the *Four Last Songs* by Richard Strauss . . . it's a connecting up with the hundreds of years of human experience . . . a sort of continuity of being which is distilled into these wonderful melodies and . . .

MB: And the message is?

Susan: It's the same message I hear as I sit on top of my favourite hill in Scotland. In the absolute silence I look at this place and it's as timeless and ancient and as perfect as it could be and I'm just a small speck here . . . I'm just part of the whole continuum.

MB: And it's alright? . . .

Susan: Yes . . . yes and it's OK.

The *Four Last Songs* – Richard Strauss, sung by Jessye Norman

---

The *Four Last Songs* by Richard Strauss are entitled: Spring, September, Going to Sleep and At Gloaming. What is particularly poignant about these songs is that Strauss died before they were heard in public and it seems also that the first performance sung by Kirsten Flagstad was nine days after his wife died.

   We are going to talk mainly about only one of the songs – Number 3 – 'Going to Sleep', but first say a little bit about 'Spring'.

Susan: It is so marvellous. There is a sort of build-up of intensity in the orchestra, dark flowing movement, something is going to happen and then this voice suddenly bursts open and there is this explosion of beautiful sound . . . she hits that high note and . . . I sort of stand there and feel as if my hair is blowing back . . . it's a kind of . . . Wow! moment within the first few bars. This is the piece I listen to when I want to connect with some intensity in myself . . . when there is something going on in me. If I want to scream or something like that . . . this is the piece of music . . . I put it on, I turn it up . . . and let rip! But it is Jessye Norman's performance in particular which does this for me.

MB: Right . . . but we turn now to the song which you have especially chosen. Interestingly you have chosen 'Going to Sleep'. What does this music mean for you Susan?

Susan: It is acceptance for me . . . it has forgiveness and a sense of acceptance especially in the violin solo in the middle . . . it is almost heaven-like for me. When I listen to this there is a sense of peace . . . a coming to terms with something and I suppose in my fantasy Strauss is saying, ''This is probably one of the last things I write. I know I'm not going to live much longer'' . . . and there is acceptance.

MB: What you are saying has parallels with the words of the songs here and it's interesting that you don't attend to the words. At the beginning the words are not so much about the subject trying to stay awake but whether he or she will accept this state of sleep? The violin comes in and gently takes the weariness of the subject and leads him or her into this wonderful deep darkness. The poem actually describes this place as the 'magic circle of night' and there is this sense of invitation and acceptance.

Susan: But it doesn't feel like darkness to me. It just feels like repose and peace. But of course there is also a little bit of hope there.

MB: Oh . . . then the wonderful sequence in the orchestra which is taken up by the voice.

Susan begins to sing it in flowing reaching leaps and there is some mild chaos of conversation and joint singing of the sequence, with waving arm movements from both of us, while following the melodic contours of the melody. All of this ends in much laughter.

MB: Yes . . . there is hope and joy there isn't there?

Susan: And there is also a bit of melancholy at the start and then it begins to move upwards in this ascending sequence and that's when it doesn't really matter, nothing matters . . . I am part of a bigger world. After the melancholy and sadness it's all going to be over. It's the acceptance of this and the transcendence of this. Everything is alright . . . I'm part of the bigger picture. When I hear this piece of music there is some comfort from the fear of dying. The music echoes for me the things I find comforting. It kind of embodies them.

MB: Of the singers who have recorded this piece Jessye Norman is the one you would choose?

Susan: She sings like James Galway plays the flute. When I first heard James Galway play I was driving a car and had to pull over. I couldn't listen to this kind of flute playing and drive . . . I had never heard that quality of sound before . . . and it's the same with Jessye Norman's voice.

MB: There is a kind of raw earthiness about this voice?

Susan: Yes, and it's very vital and gorgeous . . . what an instrument. To my mind it doesn't suit all the aspects of these songs . . . but when I'm looking for that . . . essence of life, then she's the one I want to hear. She's the one who's living it in the songs.

MB: Do you think, Susan, that when you played the flute in that competition all those years ago, which you won, you may have experienced some of that vitality in your own playing?

Susan: At my best as a player . . . yes . . . I had that voice . . . that was the sound I made when I poured my heart into it . . . full of vitality. That was always what people noticed about my playing . . . It was that passionate sexy girl caught up in that skinny 15-year-old body.

MB: You talked earlier about music in general telling you something *now*. I wonder if you could say more?

There was a great burst of laughter from Susan at this point.

Susan: That I'm a great sexy girl now? ... I'm hardly a girl. I think what I hear now in music is that vitality which I guess I now know I have. So I'm going to be one of those great old babes and I'll be sitting there at 90 and people will be saying "What a great old babe she is"! That's what I want to be!

MB: Thank you Susan.

References

Robb L (1999) Emotional musicality in infant-mother vocal affect, and an acoustic study of postnatal depression. *Musicae Scientiae*. Special Issue 1999–2000. The European Society for the Cognitive Sciences, Belgium, pp. 123–54.

PART 3

Time for Reflection

CHAPTER 13

Commonalities and differences

In the last ten chapters the interviewees have generously told us something of what music means for each of them. This is not a scientific enquiry research project, nor are the reflections in this chapter psychotherapeutic case study analyses, so how might we understand something of what we have been told? Each account has been partly autobiographical and a personal history of how the experience of listening to music has been different for each of them at different periods of their lives.

We could begin to think about these personal narratives in the categories used by EM Foster described here in Chapter 1. Have some of the interviewees seemed to hear the music like Mrs Munt who listened to the rhythmic pulse primarily, or like Helen who listened imaginatively to Beethoven's *Fifth Symphony* and pictured heroes and shipwrecks, or like Margaret who can see only the music? Somehow these broad categories do not do justice to the complexity of the experiences of music which have been presented to us. Apart from the personal experiences of music from people from different cultures, each interviewee has told us something of what it is to be that particular person, who they are and who he or she is as a person-in-relationship in the world, and how music is inextricably linked with that experience.

As has been said above, these interviews are not psychotherapeutic consultations but are in-depth conversations. The in-depth answers which have been given call for a range of interdisciplinary understandings, which in the full range of their breadth and depth are beyond the scope of this book. More comprehensive understandings would include aspects of the cognitive psychology of music, behavioural biology with special reference to short and long-term memory and infant/mother research in healthcare. All of these areas could be considered in such a discussion. However, there are territories of study already mentioned, such as the philosophy of music, developmental psychology, psychoanalytic understandings and new findings in neuroscience, from which we may start to learn more about this human experience of listening to music.

In this chapter, I will once again draw on the philosophy of music of Susanne Langer and Victor Zuckerkandl, developmental psychology in the work of Daniel Stern, psychoanalytic understandings from the work of DW Winnicott and Christopher Bollas and neuroscience and music by looking at current work by Colwyn Trevarthen and Antonio Damasio.

The 15 interviewees in this book, including the three young choristers from the Kinder Choir, have presented us with their experiences of listening to music, as did three persons from different cultures. How then can we begin to understand something of all these experiences? One method is to consider commonalities and differences, in groups and individually. We will consider these commonalities and differences under the following headings:

- active music making
- communities and music
- music in association with words
- the aesthetic experience of music and its roots in infancy
- the therapeutic practice of listening to music.

Active music making

One feature which is common to all interviewees is that apart from listening, the comtemplative mode of attending to music, they each have written of the active experience of engaging with music. Colwyn Trevarthen identifies this active aspect in his work with newborn babies and mothers. He holds the view that these active and contemplative aspects are two sides of the one growing experience of music for the human child.[1]

Starting with Will, his active engagement is in composing music itself and he has played in orchestras and small groups, as has Susan. Here the instrument is more objective, outside the body. It is interesting that Susan chose a singer for her special piece of music and noted the importance of this expression of selfhood in the voice. Dr Margaret also noted that the singing voice is an instrument which is literally built into the body and in this sense is certainly less expensive to make music with than purchasing a musical instrument for a child. Maggie noted the importance of choral singing when she was younger in that it gave her a sense of who she was in the world and a sense of her own emotionality. She now considers her psychotherapeutic practice as a kind of parallel practice of music in which she engages with musical dynamics in a psychotherapeutic conversation. She works with the contours of affect (feeling and emotion) as if they were musical lines, a duet with the client. These musical lines of the therapeutic conversation are shaped by the dynamics of crescendo, decrescendo, silence, stillness, excitement and calm. These are the same kinds of forms of feeling that Susanne Langer explores in her writings[2] and which Stern has identified in infant/mother interaction as 'vitality affects'.[3]

The other philosopher of music whose writing is called on in this book is Zuckerkandl and he maintains that music is motion in the dynamic field of tones. Psychotherapy, as Maggie describes it, could perhaps be called mental motion in the dynamic field of persons. The difference here is that psychotherapeutic dynamic motion is not with singing or musical instruments but with personal presence, silence and spoken words.

Both the Anglican priests David and Reg have sung in choirs and Reg is still active musically, singing and going on tour in his choir at the age of 100. Maeve and Dr Margaret both sing in choirs and engage actively with this experience of music. Keith has sung in choirs but also plays the cello in his University of the Third Age group. Susan has played in orchestras and chamber music groups in her career as a musician and now, interestingly, has become a counsellor and psychotherapist who knows like Maggie the dynamics of interpersonal relationships, not because she has been taught this type of interpersonal engagement in her psychotherapy training, which will have of course happened, but because she is a musician who knows about such fine dynamics of feeling. The young persons in the Kinder Choir are actively participating in music now and from their written accounts have also begun to engage reflectively with the contemplative aspect of this experience of music in their lives.

I have left Safiya, Wajiha and Roopa to the last as their active musical participation is interestingly different, coming as they do from an Eastern culture. They have never belonged to a choir in India because such a musical gathering is not part of their culture. However, as will be seen from the following discussion, one aspect of being in a choir is a sense of community and their respective cultures embody this musical aspect of human behaviour deep within their identities.

Communities and music

As has been noted above, musical communities can be choirs or orchestras, or smaller groupings such as string quartets. We will consider first the secular choir, because the interviewees as adults are engaged with this form of group singing, as is also the Kinder Choir. So that we can say more about the experience of being in a choir, a working definition is useful. A choir is a gathering of adults and/or children engaged in performing and making music together under the leadership of a conductor.

The secular choir has its beginnings in the madrigals of the sixteenth century and it developed through the rise of nationalism in Europe, whilst the religious church choir goes back to the worship in the Jewish Second Temple at Jerusalem (539 BC–70 AD).[4]

From the writings of the interviewees, being a member of a choir or orchestra is a special experience of coming together. The psychoanalyst DW Winnicott would identify such an active experience of music as an adult form of play.[5]

Staying with such analytic thinking for a moment, one might think of the choir as a metaphor for the communication within a family and even family relationships. It could be thought of as a container for interaction between the choir members, 'the children', and the conductor as the 'mother/father'. They are all engaged in a creative pleasurable activity; the children want to please 'mother/father' (as the Kinder chorister Charlotte articulated), and the conductor, 'mother/father', wants to bring out the best in the children.

They do this by directing the children authoritatively and firmly (the father aspect) and by listening carefully and responding to the flowing interpersonal dynamic between the choristers, 'children', and themselves (the mother aspect) as they are all caught up in the flowing dynamic which is music. The man or woman conductor will of course embody both the male/female aspects of the conductor. As directors of the group they have primary responsibility for 'reading' or interpreting the contours and flow of music, and the choristers have the responsibility of attending carefully to the conductor and opening their own hearts to the flow of the music and the guidance of the conductor. When this works best it is a truly joyous family moment.

From a neuroscience perspective on play, Colwyn Trevarthen describes an infant–mother dynamic of playful interaction in which a young infant responds by waving her arms as the mother sings.[6] What is notable and measurable in this scientific observation is that the infant responds by mirroring the contour lines of sound. Of further interest here is that Trevarthen describes the infant's hand and arm movements as 'conducting' the contour lines of the mother's voice. This is more than mirroring of the mother; the baby seems to start the movement, and takes charge of the starting and stopping at certain moments. Is it possible that we have in this observation the beginnings of the choir dynamic in reverse, with the baby conducting the parent sometimes?

Returning to the aspect of community in the secular choir, each choir member literally depends on the other choir members for their very existence as to the sound they make together as they sing as one voice. Reg Dean describes it accurately as a 'band of brothers'. This family aspect has been referred to above with the choir as a kind of family with a mother/father conductor. Interestingly, Reg Dean's male voice choir did have a woman conductor for some time!

As Joyce Ellis has said, a choir can attempt difficult challenging music which would be out of reach for an individual choir member who did not have years of training as a solo singer. From a community perspective, many hurdles can be overcome by cooperation with a group of like-minded people working together towards a common goal. Safiya, Wajiha and Roopa know instinctively about this aspect of community.

Susan has described the commonalities and differences in belonging to a small group of instrumentalists and belonging to an orchestra. She writes of the intimacy of the string quartet but also of the feeling of being part of a large community like an orchestra and being caught up in something greater than the individual self; something which transcends the whole group. Another aspect of commonality and difference has to do with how each interviewee has used words in answering the question 'What does music mean for me?'. We will now consider this more fully.

Music in association with words

Music itself is a non-verbal mode of communication, but apart from using words to communicate during each interview some interviewees used words in a particular way. They became an additional frame which enhanced what they were intending to communicate. They often used words as similies, something is like something else, or they included poetry in their descriptions of their music. In his book *The Rules are No Game*, Anthony Wilden[7] describes three forms of communication which he calls codes. We will use his categories of coding to further explore the words of the interviewees' conversations. Wilden's three codings of communication are:

- digital coding
- analog coding
- iconic coding.

In the digital coding of human communication words are clear about what they describe. They are the language of separate ideas and instructions. They explain discrete categories such as 'yes' and 'no' . They clarify argument or discussion. For example, legal papers and documents are written in digital language.

Analog coding communicates the senses, emotion, memory, images and music. It deals with that which has no tight boundary such as the flow of memory. Music, painting, lyric poetry and the writing of a novel would be described as flowing frames of analog coding.

Iconic coding is a combination of analog and digital coding to produce meaning. Meaning is something beyond the digital of this or that and more boundaried than that which is analog and in constant flow like lyric poetry or music. Articulating what music or poetry means therefore is an iconic communication. The interviews in this book are iconic communications.

What is particularly interesting in these interviews is that many of the interviewees have stepped sideways from music, as it were, and called on lyric poetry, poetic prose or images – analog communications – to further frame our understanding of what music means for them. Will used the words of the Psalm from *A Love Supreme* by John Coltrane, to elucidate further the meaning and experience of listening to John Coltrane's music. David used the poetic novel *Death in Venice* by Thomas Mann to frame his experience of the Adagietto from Mahler's *Fifth Symphony*. He also spoke of the imagery of the film *Death in Venice* to enrich his words. Maggie called on the poetry of Shakespeare to lend further understanding to the content of her musical experience whilst Reg used the Blake poem *The Sick Rose* to give a personal context to the second movement of Rachmaninov's *Second Piano Concerto*. Safiya and Wajiha heard music in the poetry of the Qur'an and Keith explored James Joyce's writing as a way of communicating the meaning of music for him. He also used the whole iconic multilayered experience of a Wagner opera, with sung words, acting, movement, colour and the drama of interpersonal relationships to further situate the meaning of music for him. The choristers of the Kinder Choir and Dr Margaret referred to songs which captured the iconic category of play, that is the action songs of the choir and Dr Margaret's playful memory of the song about chewing little bits of string. This was alongside her memory of the music and words of the Schubert lieder, *Die Schöne Mullerin*.

Susan, Maeve and Roopa described completely different experiences of music. They each felt that it was the music alone which touched them. It, itself, was an iconic communication which pointed towards the spiritual. None of the three of them knew the words of their chosen music. Maeve's choice of music was the South African *National Anthem* and Susan's choice was Jessye Norman singing the *Four Last Songs* by Richard Strauss. Roopa does not understand the language in which her chosen piece of Indian classical music is sung.

What might all of these different codings indicate? It is suggested here that those who moved towards words were searching and finding a flowing frame or context in which to explore and think deeply about the ebb and flow of what music *means* for them. They also needed to own something of the experience for themselves. Those who stayed with the ebb and flow of the music were and are in touch with the 'away from' and 'towards' of being itself, and that is enough and deeply satisfying for them.

Although Keith in his explorations of James Joyce was reaching further into the non-discrete indefinite flow of experience which meets up with the non-verbal frame of Roopa, Maeve and Susan, this non-verbal flowing place of shifting indefinite thought and feeling which holds the listener in wrapt reverie has sometimes been called the 'aesthetic experience'. For some listeners like Roopa and Maeve the word Spiritual is perhaps an appropriate word which they each would use, as also would Susan, but she might use a small 's'.

There is of course the risk that anything which we don't understand in a discrete or digital way we attribute to God. But the view that this non-verbal iconic experience of listening to music as having something to do with God may also have some truth in it.

This brings us to the point of asking if we can tentatively put some building blocks in place from the different disciplines from which we might view something of this ebb and flow, this non-verbal territory of flux in and of which we are all part. These building blocks of learning or the different disciplines we have looked at will be investigated more fully in the next chapter. But before that, we should consider the early place of non-verbal aesthetic experience which has been explored in some depth in the psychoanalytic writings of Christopher Bollas.

The aesthetic experience of music and its roots in infancy

Bollas writes of the mother being experienced as a process of transformation by her infant.[8] She is said to transform the infant's being in that she helps to integrate the instinctual, the cognitive and the affective states of the internal and environmental world of the baby. This desire of the infant to have this transformational experience repeated is said by Bollas to continue into adult life, and is found in the adult in his seeking after the aesthetic experience in passages of music and any great art which holds the promise of transformation for the listener or viewer. The aesthetic experience, which according to Bollas has its roots in very early infant–mother blissful engagements, is described by him as:

> A spell that holds self and other [*music*] in symmetry and solitude, time crystallises into space providing a rendezvous of self and other (text, composition, painting) that actualises deep rapport between subject and object [music]. The aesthetic moment constitutes this deep rapport between subject and object [music] and provides the person with a generative illusion of fitting with an object [*music*], evoking an existential memory.[9] [My italics in parentheses]

He goes on to write that the aesthetic experience is not something learned by the adult but is a recollection of something lived in early life, a pre-verbal mode of being in relationship when mother first processed and transformed our being in the world. All of the interviewees will have recognised this mode of aesthetic experience when they brought to mind music which was of importance for them. However, Roopa, Maeve and Susan in particular could be said to have accessed with more immediacy this flowing mode of non-verbal experience because words and cognitive language were so absent in their descriptions and almost dismissed as having no relevance for them here.

One interesting aspect of how it might be that these particular interviewees immediately moved to a non-verbal mode of engagement with music could be that according to Bollas these kinds of aesthetic experiences provide a strong sense of continuity and ongoingness that transcends memory of personal existence. This idea would be particularly meaningful for Roopa and Maeve because of their repeated experiences of disruption of environment while growing up. This desire for continuity which they missed could be said to be of significant importance for them. Susan, however, did not feel much satisfaction from continuity of existence in her relationship with her mother as an infant, but found something of this continuity for her sense of ongoing-being in music. In her successful flute playing she expressed who she was in the world and transformed herself in the process. This was the degree of importance music held for her in her early years.

According to Bollas, we *all seek* to relive this experience, this aesthetic of early transformation of our infant environment where things became beautiful and no longer uncomfortable. This was when we were held in a loving rapport, where *continuity* of being was or seemed assured in mother's embrace. We seek this still in adult life through our attaction to aesthetic experiences in art or music. These aesthetic moments hold a promise of life being transformed, for a time anyway, of it being made more comfortable and beautiful and seemingly ongoing. It would seem that for Roopa, Maeve and Susan this aspect of ongoingness or continuity has particular importance for them because of the many disruptions in their early lives. It is also interesting that music has such a particular attraction for them because unlike the other arts it unfolds in and over time. It takes time for one sound to reach another over a measurable period before we can experience what we know as music. It is therefore a fitting, directly flowing symbol of ongoingness and continuity of being which they might want to experience more immediately, rather than being sidetracked by words or images.

At this point it might be noted that all of the experiences of the interviewees have been therapeutic in the broadest sense of the word. All feel an improved sense of wellbeing in and through their listening to music. Dr Margaret, however, is the only one of the interviewees who explicitly used the word therapeutic to describe how music accompanied her from the deep sadness of loss and sorrow associated with her divorce to a place where she can look out on life with real moments of joy and now also participate in these moments. Her experience and her choice of music will be considered further here. This is because her journey through loss and grief to a more open receptive position in life with music alongside her on her journey may be an important process from which we can learn. Music in the therapeutic process is well documented in formal active music therapy but the contemplative side, or listening to music, in the process of verbal therapy is not well documented.

The therapeutic practice of listening to music

There is a special therapeutic practice called Guided Music and Imagery.[10] This is well established but the music is chosen by the therapist and years of special training over and above a training as a psychotherapist are necessary for this professional qualification. What may be possible to explore from Dr Margaret's description is how music *chosen by the client, not the therapist,* may be used as a medium of engagement in therapy between the therapist and client.

What seems to be very important from the very beginning of this discussion is the understanding that music is a condensed symbol (a flowing sounding frame with many layers), and the client has the key to any insights and meanings which emerge. Because it is such a condensed symbol, any meanings may only appear perhaps over time and the client must be in charge of not only the choice of a particular piece of music to be heard in the consulting room but also the pace between the choosing of different pieces of music to be listened to. This process will take time and a piece of music may be a flowing frame of multilayered meaning which may take weeks or months for the client to slowly uncover assisted by the therapist.

Dr Margaret's experience tells us of her therapeutic journey through music and of the sense of personal continuity that this therapeutic musical process held for her. Any formal use of shared listening to music in therapy must be sensitive to the above considerations because music is a very powerful medium, and the therapist must follow where the client leads and not hurry the client to uncover what she might not be ready to deal with. There must also be an awareness of the client's readiness to move on to the next piece of music, the next condensed symbol, and again the client is in charge of this as well.

One might ask why such a practice of using music in the consulting room in this way is not more widespread. Part of the answer must be that until now we quite literally did not know enough about what might be going on when music was introduced into the word-based context of the consulting room. The power of music, the depth of the condensed symbol and the need to move slowly and carefully would instil much caution in the approach of any therapist wanting to engage with such an unknown medium. With the coming together of the different disciplines of music, psychology, psychotherapy and neuroscience we are in a better place and on firmer ground to move forward with appropriate research.

Any formal model of practice of using music as a shared reflective medium in the consulting room does need more research, but Dr Margaret's account of the therapeutic effect of her contemplation of the meaning of her three pieces of music may do much to inform any such further enquiry. As has been said earlier, this book does not set out to analyse the listener's music as a psychotherapeutic case study, so there will be no personal direct interpretation *from me* on Dr Margaret's account of her journey. It will be presented as information on the therapeutic process at work.

Her first therapeutic piece was the Bach *Double Violin Concerto*. Acccording to Dr Margaret she first felt contained and soothed by this piece. She next was aware of beautiful, serene, creative communication and conversation between the two violins. After some time she found that she was drawn to the Englishness of Delius' music, in particular, *The First Cuckoo in Spring*, a sign perhaps of literally something new happening alongside her own interpretation that she was beginning to re-establish her roots as an 'English country girl at heart'. In other words something of her own deep sense of personal identity was stirring. The last pieces by Britten are interestingly unaccompanied, a reaching out on her own perhaps. She also now listens to jazz which she describes as being in touch with the daring, risky part of her.

All the phrases which she herself uses to describe the pieces she chose could perhaps be understood as titles of condensed symbols of thought and feeling. These described how she engaged with others and her world in general during her journey from a place of deep sorrow and loss to a place of light and joy. She has put down signposts as it were on her journey. These may or may not be the same signposts on any other person's musical journey, but what is interesting is that they each point to a condensed area or inner territory associated with thought and feeling which could be worked with in the consulting room. Music, a non-verbal process, could quickly pinpoint these inner areas and assist the therapeutic process

The first signpost for Dr Margaret could be called the need for *Containment and Continuity*. The next one described her need for communication which had *Gentleness and Mirroring* about it. Both these signposts were articulated by her in her description of what the Bach *Double Violin Concerto* meant for her and how she felt held and soothed by listening to it. The third signpost could be called the emergence of *A Tentative Sense of Self*. This pointed to the re-emergence of a well-grounded sense of identity – who she really was. The fourth signpost could be called *Looking Outwards to the Beauty of the World*. The natural world became beautiful again for her. This was supported by her choice of Delius' *The First Cuckoo in Spring*. It is very interesting that her fifth signpost might have been named *Being Unaccompanied*. She enjoyed at this stage the unaccompanied, different but enjoyable sounds of Benjamin Britten during her journey along this pathway. Her last signpost could have been named *A Sense of Joy*. Here she describes fun, joy and a sense of daring in her introduction to the world of jazz. She indeed had made a therapeutic journey and she herself has been a signpost for further research.

References

1   Trevarthen C (1999) Musicality and the intrinsic motive pulse: evidence from human psychobiology and infant communication. *Musicae Scientiae*, Special issue 1999–2000. The European Society for Cognitive Sciences of Music, Belgium, p. 160.
2   Langer S (1951) *Philosophy in a New Key*. Harvard University Press, Cambridge, Mass., p. 193.
3   Stern D (1995) *The Interpersonal World of the Infant*. Basic Books, New York, pp. 156–161.
4   Grout DJ and Palisca C (2001) *A History of Western Music*. WW Norton and Co, USA.
5   Winnicott DW (1989) Playing and culture. In: C Winnicott, R Shepherd and M Davis (eds) *Psychoanalytic Explorations*. Harvard University Press, Cambridge Mass., p. 205.
6   Trevarthen C (2002) *Musical Identities*. RAR McDonald, DJ Hargreaves and D Miell (eds) Oxford University Press, Oxford, p. 24.
7   Wilden A (1987) *The Rules are No Game*. Routledge and Kegan Paul, London, p. 222.
8   Bollas C (1987) *The Shadow of the Object*. Columbia University Press, New York, p. 14.
9   Bollas C (1993) The aesthetic moment and the search for transformation. In: P Rudnytsky (ed.) *Transitional Objects and Potential Spaces*. Columbia University Press, New York, p. 40.
10 Guided Music and Imagery is a course at Melbourne University Australia in which specifically sequenced classical music programmes are used to stimulate and sustain a dynamic unfolding of inner experiences.
    More information can be obtained from www.music andimagery.org.au.

CHAPTER 14

'Away from' and 'towards'

This chapter will try to place where we have been, where we are now and where we are going in our understanding of what music means for us.

Where we have been

In the last chapter we found out something of what music means for the interviewees in terms of commonalities and differences. Reference was made to the philosophy of music, developmental psychology, psychoanalytic thinking and neuroscience, which were identified in earlier chapters as possible areas of learning which could be associated with musical experience. What seems to be clear now is that in order to understand better what music means for us an interdisciplinary approach is required. We need therefore to identify areas of linkage between these disciplines. Under the heading of 'Where we are now', this chapter will attempt to only begin this enquiry and look at what one particular piece of music means for the author. Having made some linkages with the different disciplines, the last part of the chapter will address 'Where we are going'. In this part areas of research will be identified which would be best served by an interdisciplinary approach.

Where we are now

The area we are working in here could be called non-verbal in the sense that until now many of the ideas have not been brought together before in this way. As we have seen, the use of symbols helps towards the clarification of such non-verbal or pre-verbal territories of the human mind. The symbol of a flowing river eddying in pools could describe the eternal movement of music which we encounter. There is ebb and flow 'away from' and 'towards', but also movement forward, a current within water itself.

The philosophy of music, neuroscience associated with music, the structure of the feeling brain, understandings from psychoanalysis and developmental psychology could all be thought of as stepping stones on which we position ourselves to view this flowing river of music which laps around our ankles. At special aesthetic moments we seem to enter the flow but find a place on which to stand again as we reflect on our experience. So far our stepping stones have been very separate except for neuroscience and the active side of music which have come together in the work of Trevarthen and others working in the field of music and infant–mother communication.[1] This chapter will be a tentative attempt to provide further bridges or links between these two stepping stones and all the other stepping stones, so that we can better view the pools and eddies of the river of music and perhaps understand better how we can go with the flow of it as listeners and perhaps use some of its power appropriately. The first important bridge to make is between the stepping stones of the philosophy of music and findings in neuroscience. This is because these particular stepping stones reach deep into the river and are concerned not only with the motion of music but with the motion of life itself.

The philosophy of music and neuroscience

From Zuckerkandl's thinking on the philosophy of music we learn that there is a deep flowing motion of 'away from' and 'towards', an ebb and flow in the tones of music themselves. He then writes that tonal motion is a kind of mental motion, not bodily motion. It is a motion without a material underpinning and without a specific location in space. It is just itself in motion.[2] He also notes that we are reluctant to acknowledge that there is the phenomenon of self-motion, pure life motion

This pure life motion can be thought of as a deep flowing 'away from' and 'towards' which moves in through and beneath all things, permeating all things. Zuckerkandl names this dynamic movement *emotion*. (This is a very particular meaning of this word and not to be confused with the more general term 'emotions' which we use as interchangeable with feelings.) To hear music for Zuckerkandl is to hear this emotion, to hear this kind of self-motion. This self-motion would be the deepest layer of this non-verbal place, the deepest stratum in which all feeling and physical movement are rooted.[3]

But to make a further link with neuroscience we turn to the writing of Damasio in his book *Looking for Spinoza*. Here he writes most interestingly of the development of the brain. He uses the analogy of a tree. The base of the brain he calls the place of *emotion*, the basic movement of life. (He uses this word in the same particular way that Zuckerkandl does.) He defines this *emotion*, this basic movement of life, as the approaching or withdrawal of the entire organism and sees all life forms as governed by this dynamic.[4] This would be a direct link with Zuckerkandl's writing[3] on 'away from' and 'towards' as the dynamic motion or *emotion* of life itself.

Damasio goes on to describe what *is* in motion here at the base of the brain. He writes that there is the motion of 'away from', and 'towards' in the chemical and mechanical components which seek homeostasis or balance. Other automatic regulators of life in the lowest branches of this tree of the brain are basic reflexes, and the immune system. The middle level branches of this brain system are concerned with pain and pleasure behaviours and these go into action when the organism reacts to impingement or sickness of one kind or another. The next higher level of branches deals with drives and motivations and the top branches are what Damasio calls emotions proper. They are the big feeling areas of joy, sorrow, fear, pride, shame and sympathy.[5]

The linkages therefore between Zuckerkandl's philosophy of music and Damasio's neuroscientific explanation of the brain system is at a level to do with the dynamic of 'away from' and 'towards', which both disciplines agree is the deep flowing frame of life itself which seeks not only survival but wellbeing. It also permeates all other later processes. We now have some scientific evidence for Zuckerkandl's thinking.

We will now add another discipline or stepping stone to the river, that of developmental psychology.

The philosophy of music, neuroscience and developmental psychology

Daniel Stern contributes this new stepping stone, as it were, with what he describes as 'vitality affects'. These he first identifies in the growing infant.[6] They are movements of rushing, fading, crescendo, decrescendo, fleeting explosions, serene movements, and these are *ways* of expressing sadness and/or joy. These 'vitality affects'. are to do with intensity, urgency, or lack of it, of the feeling shape or contour. They are called 'background emotions' by Damasio to distinguish them from feelings proper. But they could be said to set the scene for feelings proper.

At this point there is another link to the philosophy of music in the thinking of Susanne Langer. In her thinking on music these 'background emotions' or 'vitality affects' are described by her as *forms of feeling*, as we have noted earlier. She writes of them as to do with texture and contour, the excitement of crescendo in music or the serenity and calm of a slow-moving passage of notes and phrasing in music. The complexity of trying to come to grips with what the experience of music is and how we experience it is becoming clearer. But where do we now stand?

We now have linkages between three stepping stones of the disciplines of the philosophy of music, neuroscience and developmental psychology, each contributing something different but also overlapping. These experiences are real and measurable so we are beginning very slowly to know more precisely about what music might mean for us.

If the reader can bear it, there is one further process of linkage which is important in this interdisciplinary exercise of seeing where we are in our understanding of this experience of what music means for the listener. This last linkage, the core of the book, is between the brain and *how* we process the experience of listening to music. We will turn to Langer, Damasio, and the psychoanalytic writings of Christopher Bollas for this final exploration.

In her book *Philosophy in a New Key*, Susanne Langer explores further the forms of feeling which still feed on the basic stratum of dynamic flow. However, she understands the listener's experience of music, as if by some kind of projection by him into music. The listener somehow projects from his brain into the music he is listening to.[7] How this projection takes place is not clear but Damasio goes some way to unravel this process and make it more understandable.

He writes that feelings are perceptions but the shapes, vitality affects, aural in music (or visual in the case of a painting), associated with these feelings have their origin within the person experiencing the piece of music or painting. The characteristics of this outside object, music or painting correspond to the characteristics of the original object in the brain/body. These characteristics form a kind of reflective frame.

Damasio calls this outside object, the painting or the passage of music, the 'emotionally competent object' because it resonates with the shape and structural characteristics of the original object in the mapping of the brain. So there is what he calls a correspondence between them. However, he makes it clear that the *feelings* and the events at the origin of this perception are well *inside* the body rather than *outside* it.[8] It is only the structural frame which is reflected, not the particular fine-grained feelings. The particular feelings are therefore not in the music but in the person who is experiencing the music. It is only the vitality affects or forms of feeling which are in the music *and* the listener. These would be experienced as corresponding exactly.

We turn to the fourth discipline of psychoanalysis which will further contribute to Damasio's understanding of the experience of listening to music. The psychoanalytic writing of Christopher Bollas on music as a transformational medium will complete this initial exploration of the experience of listening to music.

The philosophy of music, neuroscience, developmental psychology and psychoanalytic thought

This last stepping stone gives some explanation as to why and how it is that we retain in the brain the feelings and feeling shapes from earlier in our lives and then project these shapes and contours of feeling into music. As we have said above, we are said to encounter this material when we listen to and experience music beyond early childhood. But the questions of why and how this should be so requires some further explanation.

Why this is so will be considered first and then we will turn to how the process of listening to music itself unfolds. We will use simple diagrams to try and clarify this process.

Why do we retain shapes and feelings in the brain from infancy?

One answer to this question is provided by Christopher Bollas.[9] He suggests that we are seeking transformation of the unintegrated parts of the self. Most of who we are is well enough integrated so that we function in the world appropriately, but there are aspects of who we are which often have to do with strong feelings which are not well integrated. These feeling parts of the brain, in the inner feeling self, have a form, shape and texture and we resonate with these corresponding shapes and textures while listening to a passage of music which we find really important for us. This area is often pre-verbal, that is, from our infancy. If it was not, we would be able to think clearly and put words to our feelings, understand clearly what was going on and not need a medium of transformation.

In this pre-verbal engagement of the infant with his mother, Bollas writes that the infant's experience of his mother is as if she is an apparition whose presence and attention dissolves distress in that she makes the child more comfortable and also feeds him.[9] The state of the infant is transformed from discomfort to comfort by being changed, emptiness becomes fullness and the feeling of continuity is introduced by feeding regularly. In these ways mother transforms the infant's internal and external reality. Most importantly, however, 'continuity of being' is established and maintained. In other words, the baby learns that life is ongoing and the beginnings of trust in mother and the outside world is introduced. But what has this to do with the adult or older child listening to music? How do we make this link?

When we listen to music we literally take something in, in through our ears. Further to this, when we listen with attention as an infant does while feeding, we are held in an experience of reverie or deep rapport with a passage of music and we are not continuously in a thinking mode, rather like a baby. In this subjective experience, for the older person, thinking is suspended and experienced as somehow out there in the music or painting. This is similar to the young infant's experience of mother; the apparition who transforms our being in the world comes to us from outside.

As has been pointed out earlier in this chapter, Bollas holds the view that the aesthetic experience of listening to music is not learned by us as adults but is an 'existential recollection' of *how* we were handled by our mother or first carer and *how* our being was transformed by them and our fears of hunger and emptiness were dissolved and assuaged.

This would be supported by Damasio's thinking that we experience the shapes and contours of music deep within our body, the felt memory. This felt memory then connects with the feelings in the higher levels of the brain and we experience them as *specific feelings* of, for example, being held securely, lovingly cared for, or just feeling good inside. We can experience the felt memory of negative feelings as well, most notably that of feeling alone and frightened when, for example, mother is absent.

Eventually for the infant, words appear in the interchanges between mother/carer and child and the state of just 'being' gives way more often to the more active state of 'doing'. This then becomes integrated into the experience of thinking. However, because we continue to grow we also continue to search for that something further to make us feel complete and replete as we did in the good enfolding experiences we had as infants with mother. In other words we search for wellbeing. Areas we look to for a repetition of these experiences are music, art or religious experience. Any of these hold the hope of further transformation. This might answer why we look to the arts for such an experience.

We will now consider how this process unfolds in particular aesthetic moments. What is being described here would not apply to the length of a symphony, only for a particular significant passage of music. This longer exploration of the experience of listening to music could be called narrative listening. In this longer exploration of the experience of music, a condensed emotional story could be said to unfold for the listener. It may have several aesthetic moments in it, but any interdisciplinary research into episodic listening in developmental psychology, that is listening for longer periods of time, and its linkage with neuroscience, is still at an early stage. We just do not know enough to apply the process described below to longer passages of music.

This lack of hard scientific knowledge, however, should not preclude the careful search for more understanding of an individual's experience of such longer narrative musical experiences in the therapeutic consulting room. What is learned here could inform and contribute to neuroscientific research in an interdisciplinary enquiry in this area.

The listening process described below, however, happens over fractions of moments in time. Bollas has written on the *aesthetic moment* and the fact that we are dealing with such a short passage of time must be kept in mind.

How the momentary process of listening to music unfolds

We have been exploring quite complex processes and a diagrammatic outline might summarise and clarify this thinking (*see* pp 151–2). The unfolding process is described here as broadly therapeutic in that we are assumed to be feeling better at the end of the listening experience than we felt before it.

The process of listening to music unfolds

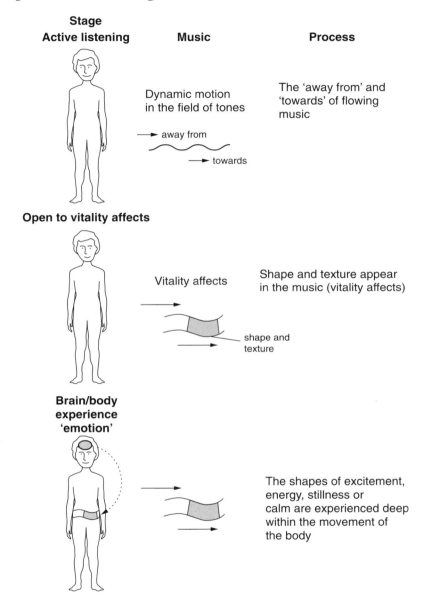

The first stage is Active listening, that is listening with attention. Here the listener is aware of the musical encounter. The second stage is Vitality affects and these are the shapes of excitement, crescendo, decrescendo, etc. as they happen in the music. The third stage describes how these vitality affects are experienced in the brain/body, i.e. the sensation of movement – 'emotion'.

Diagram continued

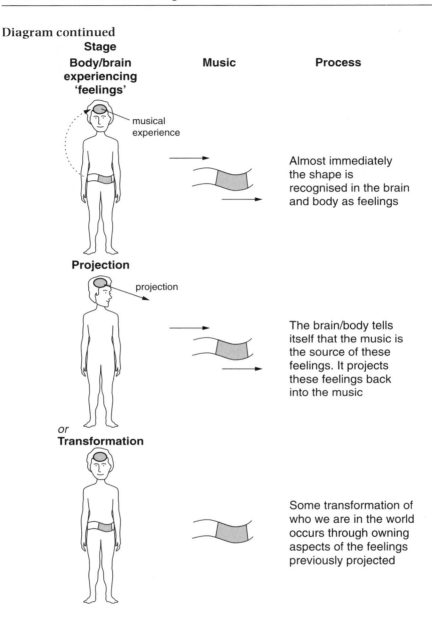

Stage

Body/brain experiencing 'feelings'	Music	Process

musical experience

Almost immediately the shape is recognised in the brain and body as feelings

Projection

projection

The brain/body tells itself that the music is the source of these feelings. It projects these feelings back into the music

or
Transformation

Some transformation of who we are in the world occurs through owning aspects of the feelings previously projected

The fourth stage describes the connection in the brain with fine-grained feelings – joy, sadness, dejection, etc.

The fifth stage is Projection. This is a mysterious concept. Projection is the disowning of feeling(s) and pushing them out into the music. This process, however, isn't an issue for us if the feeling or feelings involved are acceptable to us, like joy or happiness. We accept these feelings and do not notice the process. We project them partly into the music, experience them and the process doesn't bother us. However, if the feelings are unpleasant they become unacceptable. Unacceptable feelings are projected, pushed out, into the music and left there. The kinds of feelings which might be deemed unacceptable are, for example, vengeful feelings or despairing feelings. One then tells oneself that these feelings belong to music alone.

The last stage deals with transformation. Here one recognises the unacceptable feelings as belonging to oneself and feels transformed somewhat by these aesthetic moments.

Some further thoughts on the process of transformation

Although the process of transformation takes fractions of a second, the transformation of who we are in the world may be for a shorter or longer time. If our transformation has been for a shorter time, our mood has changed perhaps from sadness to joy on listening to a beautiful passage of music, as if mother had somehow made our world a better place, as Bollas has suggested.

I would like to consider an aspect of the longer lasting type of transformation. This is when the passage of music carries more than one feeling at the same time. Reg spoke of this with reference to Rachmaninov's *Second Piano Concerto*, where great beauty is linked with tragedy in Reg's experience. David's experience of the Adagietto from Mahler's *Fifth Symphony*, where the two feelings experienced are great beauty and great loss, is another example. This longer-lasting transformation involves taking back what has been projected into music and owning these uncomfortable feelings.

I would like to explore this kind of transformation process in a passage chosen by myself in an attempt to illustrate this particular frame of experience. The piece of music is the Dance of the Knights from Prokofiev's ballet *Romeo and Juliet*. I will briefly describe the piece and then explore the process of my own experience of it.

This piece comes during the masked ball where the warring families of Montagues and Capulets have mingled. The music of the Dance of the Knights starts with a strong powerful tonic/dominant (doh/soh) figure in the bass of the orchestra. This is the platform for a simple arpeggio figure (doh/me/soh) which is characterised by huge octave leaps, the doh/me/and soh stretching over the boundary of a single octave into the next one. The repeated bass figure underpins these wide interval leaps. The music for me is strong and powerful, with more than a hint of menace and violence. However, these tonal shapings can also be heard as exuberant, ebullient and energetic. This music carries for me both the nature of the negative and positive, both in its content and shaping of melody.

Langer has said that music can carry more than one feeling at the same time and this particular music is an appropriate example for me. I will refer to the process above to explore the experience in more detail. This of course is only one kind of such transformation.

A transformation process in the Dance of the Knights from *Romeo and Juliet*

Active listening: The first thing I notice is the 'away from' and 'towards' in the repeated tonic/dominant bass notes. Next the melodic arpeggio leaps accentuate not only 'away from' and 'towards' but upward and downward as well. This accentuated movement is heard from all around, above and below as well as horizontally.

Vitality affects: The shapes and textures of excitement and energy appear in the music.

Brain/body experience – 'emotion': The power of the swooping movement is felt throughout my body. I want at least to move my arms and also my feet.

Body/brain experience – 'feelings': Here I feel thrilling excitement, exhilaration, energy and power, but also a hint of menace and violence.

Projection: If I project the above feelings into the music I would be left with little or nothing after the performance. I am happy to keep the thrilling exhilaration but less happy to own the menace and violence. I could split this negative part off and tell myself that it's in the music and story. But as Bollas says, these powerful experiences are not first introduced in adulthood. We know about them from early life. So how do I know about feelings of violence?

My own early life was characterised by much disruption when my mother was in hospital for a year from when I was six months old. In psychoanalytic thinking it could be that my internal infant-self knows about this rage. I know about such violent feelings since they belong to me!

Transformation: If I can own this unpleasant part of me and not project it out there into the music, as if it has nothing to do with me, I am somewhat transformed and I can live more easily with these negative feelings. I don't need to deny them in real life. I can think about them and have room to process them. But how do I do this?

I do it by reflection. I know where these feelings come from in childhood, but I can reflect, as an adult, that a childish response of rage would not be appropriate here and I *can* manage these strong feelings better as an adult. In this way, these negative feelings are better integrated into my personality and I am somewhat transformed. When I hear this music again I know where to put these strong feelings; I can place them better as belonging to infancy and they don't have the intensity of power *over* me that they did when I first heard this piece.

Having explored a little of what music means for me, we will now look at the research scene and try and see, perhaps dimly, the way forward.

Where we are going

Research

There is much cognitive research done on music and its effect on our brains but very little on music and our feelings except for Damasio's writing on the adult experience of listening and the writing of Jaak Panksepp,[10] another neuroscientist whose work I discovered too late to be included in this book. This lack of research on music and feelings could be because until now there hasn't been the interdisciplinary work undertaken in this field. Notable exceptions are Colwyn Trevarthen, Stephen Malloch and Louise Robb who are looking at the infant/mother frames of communication which include feelings.[1,11,12]

Looking at the wider field of cognitive research, one of the most interesting examples detailed in the M.I.N.D. Institute on the Internet is *The Mozart Effect*,[13] in which it was found that college students who listened to the Mozart *Sonata for Two Pianos in D Major* (K448) had short-term enhancement of their spatio–temporal memory reasoning.[14] This means that they improved in the area of making a mental image and thinking ahead in space and time. Further to this, a study in 1997 with three-year-olds who were given piano lessons for six months showed long-term spacio-temporal reasoning enhancement. More research is continuing in this field. The list of examples of cognitive research could go on. However, as pointed out above, interdisciplinary research on music and feelings is thin, so far. If we knew more about linkages between such fields as music, philosophy of music, cognitive psychology, psychoanalysis and neuroscience, not only might we be able to understand better the experience of listening to music but we might also be able to address some of the more irritating facets of our urban life.

One of the common results of the dearth of research on music and feelings is that we are plagued by music at every turn. It is played in pubs, restaurants, banks, airports, department stores, hospitals, etc. If there was more interdisciplinary research which would target the consumer appropriately, we would be spared a lot of irritating noise. At the moment it seems that what we are forced to listen to is the choice of the management which chooses the music to be heard on the assumption that it knows best for us. Management assumes it knows what we feel and how to change our feelings, which really is quite a wrong assumption.

There is an organisation called 'Pipe down'[15] which campaigns against such mindless dissemination of music, particularly piped music. Their research was originally commissioned by the Royal National Institute for the Deaf (1998) as deaf people have particular difficulty in unwanted irritating music as it interferes with any hearing aids they might be using. The National Opinion Poll (NOP) research findings were as follows: 34% of people hate piped music anywhere, 30% like it and 36% are indifferent. Even this broad research does not give any basis for the noise pollution we suffer every day in our high streets, hospitals, banks, etc.

I myself have experienced much irritation in a hospital waiting area in which I might have been expected to be helped to feel calm. In this case it was piped music from Radio 1 which was heard throughout the hospital waiting areas. I asked politely for it to be turned down but I was glad when it was turned off with an apology. The biggest problem is the assumption that everyone will like this music. It is meant to 'cheer you up'. People are not being annoying deliberately. It is really a lack of knowledge and understanding.

Another real problem of course is people playing *their* music in the garden in the summer or leaving their windows open on a hot day while they are playing their favourite music which is also disturbing people all around. I'm sure these people would not enjoy Beethoven's *Fifth Symphony* thundering at them whilst they were sunbathing in the garden! But maybe that's an assumption too on my part. Research into music and feelings is much needed so that it doesn't just rely on personal preference. Another area of research which is much needed is music in therapy, and we will now consider this.

Research on music in word-based therapy

Apart from formal music therapy (active playing) in which there is much ongoing research, listening to passages of music as part of word-based therapy is another area which would benefit from research. Because music is a condensed symbol (condensed because it contains layers of feeling), my own thinking is that it could be used sparingly and occasionally in an otherwise word-based therapeutic frame of work.

The particular advantage of using music in this context is that it is essentially non-verbal, and because of this it has the capacity to contain pre-verbal material in its shapes and contours of melody and harmonic texture. It is suggested here that new neural connections and pathways in the brain can be made through careful therapeutic holding by the therapist. Therapeutic holding is a mental holding of the psychodynamic process in which the therapist's very presence and mode of supportive engagement seeks to repair something of the client's early dysfunctional neural connections.

These potential new neural connections can be supported and sustained by the chosen music as well as the therapist's presence. The changing choice of music will further inform the process of recovery indicated by the journey Dr Margaret described in Chapter 10. Further verbal work with the therapist will lead to insight and understanding for the client. This work will not be *giving* the client insight but is patiently awaiting the connections in the brain to be made and the client's insight to be discovered. It is hoped that more research can be done on this as music is quickly able to be in touch with the layers of feeling and experience which are early and pre-verbal and therefore not available to words only.

One important area in music and therapy is that of autism. Music therapy is widely used in the treatment of autism, but if there is an assumption that there is no sense of self with which to work then the aspect of the contemplative side of music will not be considered important. I would question this assumption as I myself have been involved in a form of therapy with music in the treatment of some autistic young people.[16] The journey towards interpersonal engagement with an autistic young person was as follows.

First, there was active music playing with both of us improvising together. Then came listening to what had been played by us on the tape recorder (the contemplative side). Next came drawing by the client so that a frame of feeling and action was presented and shared between both of us. The sharing was partly verbal in that I attempted to understand the frame and the feelings portrayed in the drawing in words. (The young people were either silent or had limited language.) This method had some encouraging results. But we look to further work in neuroscience and developmental psychology to inform any further work of this nature.

We have now looked into the future of where we might go in terms of research into music and feelings. It is an exciting prospect but, as Damasio warns, we must beware of explorations that rely on data from one single level or, for that matter, one single discipline. We must share our knowledge so that we have more stepping stones of understanding. This is only a beginning of understanding what the experience of music means for us.

References

1 Trevarthen C (1999) Musicality and the intrinsic motive pulse: evidence from human psychobiology and infant communication. *Musicae Scientiae*. Special Issue 1999–2000. The European Society for Cognitive Sciences, Belgium, pp. 155–211.

2 Zuckerkandl V (1956) *Sound and Symbol*. Bollingen Series XLIV. Princeton University Press, Princeton, p. 142.

3 Zuckerkandl V (1956) *Sound and Symbol*. Bollingen Series XLIV. Princeton University Press, Princeton, p. 149.

4 Damasio A (2003) *Looking for Spinoza: joy, sorrow and the feeling brain*. Heinemann, London, p. 30.

5 Damasio A (2003) *Looking for Spinoza: joy, sorrow and the feeling brain*. Heinemann, London, p. 37.

6 Stern D (1973) *The Interpersonal World of the Infant*. Basic Books, New York, pp. 156–61.

7 Langer S (1951) *Philosophy in a New Key*. Harvard University Press, Cambridge, MA, p. 51.

8 Damasio A (2003) *Looking for Spinoza: joy, sorrow and the feeling brain*. Heinemann, London, p. 91.

9 Bollas C (1993) The aesthetic moment and the search for transformation. In: PL Rudnytsky (ed.) *Transitional Objects and Potential Spaces*. Columbia Univesity Press, New York, pp. 40–49.

10 Panksepp J (1998) *Affective Neuroscience: the foundations of human and animal emotions*. Oxford University Press, New York.

11 Malloch S (1999) Mothers and infants and communicative musicality. *Musicae Scientiae*. Special Issue 1999–2000. The European Society for Cognitive Sciences, Belgium, pp. 29–58.

12 Robb L (1999) Emotional musicality in infant–mother vocal affect, and an acoustic study of postnatal depression. *Musicae Scientiae*. Special Issue 1999–2000. The European Society for Cognitive Sciences, Belgium, pp. 123–154.

13 Gordon Shaw (1993) *The Mozart Effect*. www.mindinst.org.
14 Gordon Shaw (2003) *Keeping Mozart in Mind* (2e). Academic Press, New York.
15 PIPEDOWN The Campaign Against Piped Music. P.O. Box 1722, Salisbury SP4 7US. Tel: 01980 623945.
16 Butterton M (1991) *Music in the Pastoral Care of Emotionally Disturbed Children*. PhD Birmingham University.

Further reading

Cozolino L (2002) *The Neuroscience of Psychotherapy: building and rebuilding the human brain*. WW Norton & Company, New York and London.
Shore AN (2003) *Affect Regulation and the Repair of the Self*. WW Norton & Company, New York and London.

Glossary

Affect: Feeling.

Attunement: To bring into accord or agreement.

Arpeggio: The notes of a musical chord, e.g. C–E–G played one after the other either upwards or downwards.

Basal ganglia: Groups of neurones or nerve cells beneath the outer part of the brain, the cerebral cortex. These groups of neurones play an important role in processing and carrying out complex emotions.

Brain stem: The control trunk of the brain situated at the top of the spinal cord. It is filled with neurones which perform basic tasks.

Cerebral cortex: The outer layer and uppermost part of the brain. It is the control or executive area of the dynamic, integrated whole brain.

Chord: A group of three or more musical tones sounding together.

Cognitive: Knowing as distinct from feeling.

Counterpoint: A musical device in which the composer writes more than one melody to be played at the same time.

Diatonic scale: The pattern of tones and semi-tones used as the bedrock of Western music. In written music it extends to eight notes above or below the first note, i.e. in the scale of C major it would be C, D, E, F, G, A, B, C', the last C' being one octave or eight notes higher in pitch.

Doh: The first note in the diatonic scale written in sol-fa. Sol-fa is a way of writing the notes of the scale. It is used to teach children about the idea of a scale in music. Knowledge of written music is not necessary in order to understand sol-fa. It is in ascending order: doh, re, me, fah, soh, lah te, doh' over the span of the octave, i.e. eight notes of the diatonic scale.

Dominant: The soh note or the fifth degree of the diatonic scale. It is next in dynamic importance to the tonic note. This means that its movement 'away from' the last sounded note and its pull 'towards' the next sounding note is of less intensity than the dynamic power exerted by the tonic note on the tones of the scale in a musical passage.

Dynamic: In energetic motion with a tone or tones in music or with active mental motion with another person.

Dynamic field: *In music*: The 'away from' and 'towards' motion of tones within a passage of music. There will also be a sense of completion or return within a whole piece of music.
In psychotherapy: The 'away from', 'towards' and 'return ' in a new way within the mental dynamics of the relationship between client and therapist.

Dynamic patterning: The active motion within the form or shape of a group of tones in music, and also for the listener or performer to be mirroring this musical shaping within his or her mind. For example, the pattern of feelings in the mind can seem to correspond to the flowing pattern in a passage of music.

Emotion: Generally speaking this word is loosely interchangeable with feeling or feelings. In this book the meaning is confined to movement in terms of feeling.

Feeling: In this book, this word is used as a collective term or container for feelings.

Feelings: Particular sensitivities in the mind and body which may alter one's mood. They can also be described as fine-grained nuances of felt experience. One can experience several feelings at once.

Field: A subject of study and also an area in which a force is effective.

Field of tones: The sounding context of music in which the dynamic of 'away from' and 'towards' operates.

Forms of feeling: The dynamic shapes which frame feeling or feelings, for example, rushing, expectant, hesitant, etc.

Ghazals: Classical poetry of India which is often sung. It is a narrative form of lyric poetry.

Leitmotif: A recurring passage or theme in music associated with a person, situation or thought.

Limbic core or system: A central core processing system deep in the brain. It is a collection of structures around the brain stem and important in emotional behaviour and memory of events.

Me: The third degree of the eight notes of the sol-fa scale, i.e. doh, re, me, fah, soh, lah, te, doh'.

Music: According to Zuckerkandl, and a definition which supports the thinking in this book, music is motion in the dynamic field of tones. It is also according to Langer, a symbol of the shapes of feeling in our inner mental world.

Neural pathways: These are routes in the brain and body of nerve cells.

Opera: A drama set to music in acts. It is performed by singers and instrumentalists.

Octave: An interval formed by the first note and its title name eight notes above e.g. C to C′ (eight notes above). The notes in between would be: D, E, F, G, A, B.

Projection: In this book, projection means the unconscious pushing away of feelings into music and responding to them as if music is their only location.
In psychoanalysis and psychotherapy: It is a phenomenon in which the feelings we deny in ourselves are unconsciously projected into another person. This other person can be the analyst or therapist. We then relate to these denied feelings which we ourselves have. We may claim that the analyst or therapist is furious with us when in fact we are denying that we are furious with an aspect of ourselves.

Psychoanalysis: A psychological treatment which aims to bring unconscious material in the patient's mind into conscious thought where it is then investigated in the joint conversation between analyst and patient.

Psychodynamic: A mental process in which the mind is regarded as a phenomenon which is active as opposed to static and in relationship to aspects of the self, other persons and outside phenomena such as music or painting.

Psychodynamic psychotherapy: A psychological treatment which engages with the relationships between different parts of the client's inner world and the inner aspects of the mental world of the therapist. It aims at a good-enough inner mental state for the client in which they feel more comfortable in interpersonal relationships and there are less examples of extreme responses to others and events in the outside world.

Qur'an: This is the sacred book of Islam. In English it is the Koran.

Quwalli: Classical Indian song which was originally devotional.

Soh: The fifth degree of the eight notes of the sol-fa scale. It is in dynamic relationship with the other eight tones of the diatonic scale: doh, re, me, fah, *soh*, lah, te, doh. It is second in dynamic importance in the force field of this scale. In the diatonic scale of C major, C, D, E, F, G, A, B, C′, C is doh and G is soh.

Structures of our emotional lives: This phrase of Susanne Langer means the shapes and textures of the motion in our inner world of feeling. For example, the slow, seething, build-up of anger would be a structure in the emotional inner world of an individual.

Synaesthesia: This occurs when there is a cross-over in the senses. For example, one would be able to hear a colour. The aural has crossed over to the visual.

Tones: In this book, tones are understood to be musical notes in dynamic relationship to each other.

Tonic: The tonic or first tone of the diatonic scale. It is the anchor or most important tone of that scale. In the scale of C major, the tone C is the tonic and is in dynamic relationship with the other degrees of this scale, i.e. C, D, E, F, G, A, B, C'.

Transitional phases: Specific phases throughout life which act as bridges from one life-stage to another. For example, puberty is a transitional phase linking childhood to adolescence. Mid-life is another transitional phase linking adulthood to more mature older age.

Transitional phenomena: This is a phrase associated particularly with the psychoanalyst DW Winnicott. He first described transitional objects or transitional phenomena as those objects or phenomena used by infants to protect themselves from the fear and dread of loss of a mother and to maintain something of her presence when she was not there. Objects such as a dummy or the teddy bear would be considered as transitional objects. Winnicott also held the view that when we leave childhood and grow into adults, art, music or religion could become transitional phenomena which hold and maintain us psychologically.

Unconsummated symbol: This phrase of Susanne Langer is used by her to describe how music can symbolise the structures of our inner world. The structures of our inner world are what she calls the forms of feeling, i.e. the ways in which we experience feeling – the rushings, the expectancies – to describe our feeling experiences. But the unconsummated symbol is unconsummated because it does not fully describe the nature of the feeling itself, the fine-grained nuances of anger or joy. The nature of feeling itself belongs to the person experiencing it and is not fully symbolised in the passage of music.

Vitality affects: These are similar to the forms of feeling of Susanne Langer. They are *ways* of feeling and experiencing described by Daniel Stern, especially in relation to his observation of infant behaviour. These ways of feeling are kinetic terms such as rushing, fading away, exploding, etc.

Index